RESPONSE OF DIFFERENT SPECIES TO TOTAL BODY IRRADIATION

SERIES IN RADIOLOGY

J. Odo Op den Orth, The Standard Biphasic-Contrast Examination of the Stomach and Duodenum. Method, Results and Radiological Atlas.
1979. ISBN 90 247 2159 8

J.L. Sellink and R.E. Miller, Radiology of the Small Bowel. Modern Enteroclysis Technique and Atlas.
1981. ISBN 90 247 2460 0

R.E. Miller and J. Skucas, The Radiological Examination of the Colon. Practical Diagnosis.
1983. ISBN 90 247 2666 2

S. Forgács, Bones and Joints in Diabetes Melitus.
1982. ISBN 90 247 2395 7

G. Németh and H. Kuttig, Isodose Atlas. For Use in Radiotherapy.
1981. ISBN 90 247 2476 7

J. Chermet, Atlas of Phlebography of the Lower Limbs, including the Iliac Veins.
1982. ISBN 90 247 2525 9

B. Janevski, Angiography of the Upper Extremity.
1982. ISBN 90 247 2684 0

M.A.M. Feldberg, Computed Tomography of the Retroperitoneum. An Anatomical and Pathological Atlas with Emphasis on the Fascial Planes.
1983. ISBN 0 89838 573 3

L.E.H. Lampmann, S.A. Duursma and J.H.J. Ruys, CT Densitometry in Osteoporosis. The Impact on Management of the Patient.
1984. ISBN 0 89838 633 0

J.J. Broerse and T.J. MacVittie, Response of Different Species to Total Body Irradiation.
1984. ISBN 0 89838 678 0

RESPONSE OF DIFFERENT SPECIES TO TOTAL BODY IRRADIATION

J.J. BROERSE
Radiobiological Institute TNO
Rijswijk
The Netherlands

T.J. MACVITTIE
Armed Forces Radiobiology Research Institute
Bethesda, Maryland
USA

1984 **MARTINUS NIJHOFF PUBLISHERS**
a member of the KLUWER ACADEMIC PUBLISHERS GROUP
BOSTON / DORDRECHT / LANCASTER

Distributors

for the United States and Canada: Kluwer Academic Publishers, 190 Old Derby Street, Hingham, MA 02043, USA
for the UK and Ireland: Kluwer Academic Publishers, MTP Press Limited, Falcon House, Queen Square, Lancaster LA1 1RN, England
for all other countries: Kluwer Academic Publishers Group, Distribution Center, P.O. Box 322, 3300 AH Dordrecht, The Netherlands

Library of Congress Cataloging in Publication Data

Main entry under title:

Response of different species to total body
    irradiation.

    (Series in radiology)
    Based on a workshop organized by the Radiological
Institute TNO and the Armed Forces Radiobiological
Institute held at Rijswijk on July 1, 1983.
    Includes bibliographies.
    1. Radiation--Physiological effect--Congresses.
2. Radiation--Toxicology--Congresses. I. Broerse, J. J.
II. MacVittie, T. J. III. Nederlandse Organisatie
voor Toegepast-Natuurwetenschappelijk Onderzoek ten
behoeve de Volksgezondheid. Radiobiologisch Instituut.
IV. Armed Forces Radiobiology Research Institute (U.S.)
V. Series. [DNLM: 1. Species Specificity--congresses.
2. Whole Body Irradiation--adverse effects--congresses.
WN 620 R434 1983]
QP82.2.R3R47 1984   616.9'897   84-16647
ISBN-13:978-94-009-6050-3   e-ISBN-13:978-94-009-6048-0
DOI: 10.1007/978-94-009-6048-0

ISBN-13:978-94-009-6050-3

Copyright

TABLE OF CONTENTS

List of First Authors

Ainsworth, E.J., Biology and Medicine Division, Lawrence Berkeley
    Laboratory, Berkeley, CA 94720, U.S.A.

Barrett, Ann, The Royal Marsden Hospital, Downs Road, Sutton Surrey
    SM2 5PT, United Kingdom

Baverstock, K.F., MRC Radiobiology Unit, Harwell, Didcot, Oxon OC11
    ORD, United Kingdom

Broerse, J.J., Radiobiological Institute TNO, P.O. Box 5815, 2280 HV,
    Rijswijk, the Netherlands.

Carsten, A.L., Medical Department Brookhaven National Laboratory
    Upton, New York 11973, U.S.A.

Conklin, J.J., Armed Forces Radiobiology Research Institute, Bethesda,
    Maryland, U.S.A.

Fliedner, T.M., Department of Clinical Physiology and Occupational
    Medicine, University of Ulm, D-7900 Ulm/Donau, Fed. Rep. of
    Germany.

Kaul D.C., Science Applications, Inc., 1701 E. Woodfield Rd., Suite
    819, Schaumburg, Illinois 60195, U.S.A.

Lemaire, G., Groupe Mixte de Recherche, CEA-DRET, Fontenay-aux-
    Roses, France.

MacVittie, T.J., Experimental Hematology Department, Armed Forces
    Radiobiology Research Institute, Bethesda, Maryland 20814, U.S.A.

Seed, T.M., Division of Biological and Medical Research, Argonne
    National Laboratory Argonne, IL, 60439, U.S.A.

Smith, H., National Radiological Protection Board, Chilton Didcot,
    United Kingdom

Vriesendorp, H.M., Northwestern University, Chicago, IL, U.S.A.

Zoetelief, J., Radiobiological Institute TNO, P.O. Box 5815, 2280 HV,
    Rijswijk, the Netherlands.

RESPONSE OF DIFFERENT SPECIES TO HIGH DOSE TOTAL BODY IRRADIATION

Introduction

J.J. Broerse, Radiobiological Institute TNO, Rijswijk, The Netherlands, and T.J. MacVittie, Armed Forces Radiobiology Research Institute, Bethesda, MD, USA.

During the past decade, relatively few new studies have been initiated on the response of different species to high-dose, total-body irradiation. For information on the $LD_{50/30d}$ (the dose which produces 50 percent lethality within 30 days), one is generally referred to the older literature (e.g., Bond, Fliedner and Archambeau, 1965). Comparison of experimental data reveals considerable variations in LD_{50} values even after total-body irradiation with conventional X rays, ranging from 4 to 6 Gy in the monkey, 7.1 to 9 Gy in the rat and from 6.4 to 9 Gy in the mouse (see also Hall, 1978).

Part of the discrepancy in the LD_{50} values can possibly be attributed to inadequacies in the dosimetry procedures and exposure arrangements employed. As far as clinical experience is concerned, there is now an appreciable amount of information available about the effect of total-body irradiation as a conditioning treatment for bone marrow transplantation in patients suffering from leukaemia or aplastic anaemia. The results from different centres, including the incidence of complications such as radiation pneumonitis, are considerably different. This can partly be connected with the application of different radiation schedules: large single dose versus fractionated or protracted irradiation. In addition, it is important to compare the absolute dosimetry and the experimental arrangements. The physical aspects of total-body irradiation of the human have recently been summarized and evaluated (Broerse and Dutreix, 1982) during a workshop organized by the European Late Effects Project Group (EULEP) and the European Bone Marrow Transplant Group (EBMT).

It was felt timely to review our present knowledge on lethality in different species after total-body irradiation. A workshop on this topic was jointly organized by the Radiobiological Institute TNO and the Armed Forces Radiobiology Research Institute, and was held at Rijswijk on July 1, 1983.

The aims of the workshop were to discuss LD_{50} values for a number of mammalian species and the underlying cellular mechanisms. Main emphasis was placed on the response of larger animals including dogs, pigs, monkeys, and man after exposure to radiation of different qualities. In addition, the influence of dose rate and fractionation was discussed specifically with regard to the establishment of LD_{50} and RBE values. Since dosimetry and dose distribution are essential to evaluate the biological results obtained by different groups, these topics were covered in two separate presentations. A round table discussion on a number of specific questions was held at the end of the workshop.

The present proceedings contain the full text of the individual presentations, summaries of the comments on the individual papers and a concluding summary of the round table discussion. Special words of thanks are expressed for the financial support from the U.S. Defense Nuclear Agency and for the efficient cooperation of the secretarial staff of the Radiobiological Institute TNO.

Bond, V.P., Fliedner, T.M. and Archambeau, J. 1965. Mammalian Radiation Lethality. A disturbance in cellular kinetics. Academic Press, USA.

Broerse, J.J. and Dutreix, A. 1982. Physical aspects of total body irradiation. J. Eur. Radiotherapie, 3, 157-264.

Hall, E.J. 1978. Radiobiology for the Radiologist. Second edition. Harper and Row Publishers, USA.

Some practical aspects of dosimetry and dose specification for whole body
irradiation

J. Zoetelief, L.A. Hennen* and J.J. Broerse
Radiobiological Institute TNO, P.O. Box 5815, 2280 HV Rijswijk, The
Netherlands and *Interuniversity Institute of Radiopathology and
Radiation Protection, Leiden, The Netherlands

1. Introduction

The objectives of dosimetry and dose administration concern the
specification of the temporal and spatial distribution of the energy
deposition at a macroscopic and microscopic level. It is evident that the
experimental techniques and the required dosimetric accuracy vary
greatly depending on the application. However, the planning of an
experiment and the choice of a method of measuring and reporting
dosimetric parameters should follow certain general principles to insure
that an optimum amount of information is made available. Complete
specification of dosimetric parameters may be quite important to an
individual wishing to use radiobiological data in an attempt to establish
correlations or to test a hypothesis, and neither insufficient dose
specification nor uncertainties with respect to accuracy should limit such
efforts. Dosimetry should be considered an essential part of experimental
design before radiobiological experiments are started, since often
seemingly minor modifications may result in simplified and more accurate
dosimetry and irradiation arrangements yielding complex or unusual
radiation patterns can be avoided.

Reports on the response of different species to high dose total body
irradiation released during the past two decades show a considerable
variety in specification of the dosimetry. The varying approaches
obscure the assessment of reliable dose levels for occurrence of radiation
syndromes. The present contribution deals with dosimetric quantities
and units, methods for determining the absorbed dose and dose
distribution in phantoms including the influence of inhomogeneities. With

a simple model for the survival of bone marrow stem cells, the biological consequences of an inhomogeneous dose distribution are indicated.

2. Dosimetric quantities and units

A summary of radiation quantities, units and their domain of application is given in Table 1. The most elementary characterization of a radiation field is one in terms of the type, energy, direction and number of particles. Such a description can be made by employing the quantities fluence, fluence rate, energy fluence, energy fluence rate, and differential spectra of fluence and energy fluence (see, e.g., ICRU 1980).

Table 1

Radiation quantities, units and their domain of application

Quantity	symbol	unit old	SI	domain of application	special application
energy	E	erg	J or eV	basic description of radiation	-
fluence	φ	cm^{-2}	m^{-2}	basic description of radiation field	-
fluence rate	$\dot{\varphi}$	$cm^{-2}s^{-1}$	$m^{-2}s^{-1}$	basic description of radiation field	
exposure	X	R	$C.(kg\ air)^{-1}$	basic description of photon field	still used for calibration
kerma	K	rad	$Gy(or\ J.kg^{-1})$	basic description of fields of un-charged radiation	will most likely be used for calibration free-in-air
absorbed dose	D	rad	Gy	macroscopic description of energy imparted by radiation to matter	radiobiology, radiotherapy, will be used for calibration in-phantom
dose equivalent	H	rem	Sv	macroscopic description of energy imparted by radiation to matter weighted for the risks of the type of radiation and other dose modi-fying factors	radiation protection
quality factor	Q	-	-	risk factor for a type (and energy) of radiation	radiation protection
linear energy transfer	LET	$keV.cm^{-1}$	$MeV.\mu m^{-1}$	description of microscopic energy deposition	radiation protection and previously used for radiobiology
lineal energy	y	$keV.cm^{-1}$	$MeV.\mu m^{-1}$	description of microscopic distri-bution of energy deposition (radia-tion quality)	radiobiology

The quantity exposure is still used to describe the radiation field for X and gamma radiation from a few keV up to about a few MeV. However, in connection with the introduction of the International System of Units (SI) it was recognized that the roentgen ($1R=2.58\times10^{-4}C.kg^{-1}$ in air) is not an SI unit and has to be eliminated. Difficulties associated with the introduction of SI units for exposure will most likely lead in the future to the adoption by the standardization laboratories of the quantity kerma (in air) to characterize the photon field. The kerma is the quotient of dE_{tr} by dm where dE_{tr} is the sum of the initial kinetic energies of all the charged ionizing particles liberated by uncharged ionizing particles in a material of mass dm (ICRU 1980). The special name for the unit adopted in the SI system is the gray, symbol Gy; $1Gy=1J.kg^{-1}=100$ rad, where the rad is the old unit still used in many publications.

To predict the responses of biological objects subjected to ionizing radiation it is essential to determine the energy dissipation at a macroscopic level. This can be achieved by a specification of absorbed dose and its temporal and spatial distributions. The absorbed dose is the quotient of $\overline{d\epsilon}$ by dm where $\overline{d\epsilon}$ is the mean energy imparted by ionizing radiation to matter of mass dm (ICRU, 1980). The special name for the unit of absorbed dose is the gray. Absorbed dose is defined for both charged and uncharged particles contrary to kerma, which is only defined for indirectly ionizing radiation. For radiobiological purposes, absorbed dose is usually specified in ICRU muscle tissue (ICRU, 1977) or water.

Specification of absorbed dose is not sufficient for predicting the quantitative effects of radiation on biological specimens since equal doses of different types of radiation do not produce the same frequency or incidence of biological effects. Information should, therefore, be provided on the microscopic distribution of energy dissipation i.e. radiation quality. Attempts to account for radiation quality led first to the concept of linear energy transfer (LET) and its distributions and more recently to the microdosimetric quantities lineal energy (y), specific energy imparted (z) and their distributions (see e.g., Rossi, 1968 and ICRU, 1980).

3. Requirements for dose specification and dose delivery in radiobiology

A prerequisite for radiobiological studies is that the energy dissipation in the irradiated material be determined with a sufficient degree of accuracy and precision. Investigations in radiobiology and radiotherapy have demonstrated that differences of 10 per cent in absorbed dose can produce clearly observable variations in biological response. It has therefore been suggested that an accuracy (overall uncertainty) of less than about 5 per cent and a precision (reproducibility) of within 2 per cent is required for the determination of absorbed dose in radiobiological studies. This is a difficult task, considering the complexity of dose determination due to inhomogeneities in tissue composition and density in the biological specimen.

The irradiation of a target area (e.g., tissue, organ or animal) should be uniform. The condition for uniform irradiation is that the inevitable variation in absorbed dose throughout the volume of interest should be small enough to prevent a significant effect on the biological response considered. The criterion for uniform irradiation is a maximum ratio of 1.10 in the absorbed dose at different positions in the target volume but preferably 1.05 (ICRU, 1979). For partial body irradiations, the absorbed dose in other essential organs should be as small as practically possible, certainly restricted to levels which do not interfere with the projected course of the experiment.

A description of the irradiation conditions should comprise the geo- metrical arrangement i.e., source-to-surface distance (SSD), field size(s), uni-or multi-directional irradiation, location and dimensions of organ or animal of interest, information about scattering, attenuation, or shielding materials, (wedge) filters , etc. Furthermore, the absolute absorbed dose and relative dose distribution expressed in muscle tissue in the target volume as well as in other essential parts of the irradiated animal should be stated. The radiation quality should be specified. For X irradiations, radiation quality can be indicated by stating the tube voltage, filtration and half value layer (HVL) thickness. An indication of radiation quality can also be attained by providing information on the energy spectrum of the radiation of interest. Neutron fields are always contaminated with photons. Because of the difference in relative biological effectiveness (RBE) of these two radiation components it is necessary to separately determine the neutron and photon absorbed doses.

4. Dosimeters

Calibrated ionization chambers are commonly considered as the most practical method for dose determinations for biomedical applications. For neutron dosimetry these devices are generally made tissue equivalent to facilitate the validity of the Bragg-Gray conditions (see, e.g. ICRU,

1977). The absorbed dose can be derived from the measurement of the charge collected in the chamber after correction for ion recombination, density and composition of the filling gas and shape, composition and thickness of the chamber wall (see, e.g., ICRU, 1969 and 1977).

Calorimetry is in principle an absolute method for the determination of (total) absorbed dose requiring thermal, mechanical and electrical measurements only since eventually almost all energy dissipated in matter appears as heat (see, e.g., Gunn, 1976). However, the method is too laborious for routine use and should serve rather as a reference system for calibration purposes.

The most advantageous features of thermoluminescent dosimeters (TLD) are their small size and applicability over a wide dose range. The dose information can remain stored over relatively long time periods. The principle of use is that due to energy deposition in crystalline meaterials, electrons can become trapped at lattice imperfections. By elevating the temperature of the material the electrons can escape from their traps under the emission of visible light (thermoluminescence). The resulting glow curves can have different patterns depending on the quality of the employed radiation.

Semiconductor detectors are solid state analogs of ionization chambers, the charge carriers being electrons and holes. The use of a solid as detector material is attractive because the sensitive layer can be very thin while absorbing enough energy to give good sensitivity. Their response is not as stable as that of ionization chambers and they need to be calibrated and thoroughly investigated for specific operating conditions. For applications in neutron and photon dosimetry one should be aware of the dependence of the sensitivity on radiation energy.

Well-characterized and quantitative chemical changes in aqueous solutions (e.g., the ferrous sulphate system, Fricke and Hart, 1966) can be employed for the assessment of absorbed dose. These chemical dosimeters have the advantage that they closely approximate the density and composition of biological tissue. When enclosed in a container simulating the shape of the biological volume of interest, the reading of the dosimeter provides information about the average absorbed dose in the biological specimen. Disadvantages were the relatively high doses needed (in the order of 100 Gy) and the dependence of the sensitivity on radiation quality. Recently, more sensitive solutions have been developed for measurements in the dose range of 0.1 to 30 Gy (see, e.g., Maughan et al., 1983).

5. Secondary charged particle equilibrium (interface dosimetry)

The dissipation of energy in a medium exposed to indirectly ionizing radiation is a two step process. Photons and neutrons transfer energy to electrons and atomic nuclei, respectively, and these charged secondaries dissipate the transferred energy further by undergoing electronic collisions in the medium. The two steps of energy transfer take place at different points in the medium. Because of the finite range of the charged secondaries, often the spatial absorbed dose profile is only somewhat broadened compared to that of kerma. The shifts involved in this characteristic difference approximate to the range of the secondary charged particles. Secondary charged particle equilibrium (CPE) is the situation under which the fluence of charged particles in the immediate vicinity of the point of reference is constant (ICRU, 1977). Under conditions of CPE, kerma is equal to absorbed dose when bremsstrahlung losses are negligible. If the conditions of CPE are fulfilled the absorbed dose in a medium due to photons can be derived from the exposure. Experimental conditions are usually arranged so as to provide CPE for both the dosimeter and the specimen to facilitate accurate dosimetry and to avoid nonuniform dose distributions.

A lack of secondary charged particle equilibrium occurs at any interface between adjacent materials of significantly different atomic composition. Perturbations of CPE at these interfaces can lead to considerable differences in the energy deposition by photons and neutrons (see, e.g., Sinclair, 1969 and Broerse et al., 1968). Specific examples are the irradiation of body cavities and soft tissues enclosed by bone. Another example is the build-up of CPE at air-tissue interfaces, referred to in radiotherapy as the skin sparing effect. Similar perturbations occur for irradiations of monolayers of cells in culture flasks at the interface of the culture flask material and the culture medium (see, e.g. Sinclair 1969 for X rays and Zoetelief, 1981, for neutrons). The nonuniformity of dose at the surface of a specimen irradiated in air by indirectly ionizing radiation can be easily avoided by covering it with a layer of material approximating as closely as possible the atomic composition of the specimen and having a thickness equal to the maximum range of the secondary particles present (ICRU, 1979).

6. Dose distributions in homogeneous phantoms of different size and shape for various irradiation types and arrangements

The determination of absorbed dose at various positions in a (homogeneous) reference phantom is an essential step to assess the dose distribution in the animals actually irradiated. Furthermore, this information is of interest for testing irradiation arrangements, since it can provide insight in the dose variations due to attenuation and scattering of the primary beam.

6.1 Block-shaped phantoms of different size

The degree of dose uniformity for irradiation of acrylic plastic block shaped phantoms of different size (simulating various animals) was studied. The phantoms were irradiated in absence of scatter material with 300kV X rays and ^{60}Co γ rays according to the arrangement shown in Figure 1. The dose at a point inside a phantom is denoted as D(d, l, h), where l, d and h are the distances to the centre along the depth and length height axes, respectively.

In Table 2, the maximum to minimum absorbed dose values measured along the central depth axis are given for uni- and bilateral irradiation at various distances from the centre of a phantom to the source. Since the intensity declines with increasing distance to the source, it is evident that the dose distribution in an object is dependent on this parameter. For an isotropic point source the intensity of the radiation decreases with the inverse square of the distance to the source. For extended sources the decrease with distance is less rapidly. It can be seen from Table 2 that an increase in the source to phantom distance improves the dose distribution for unilateral irradiations.

10

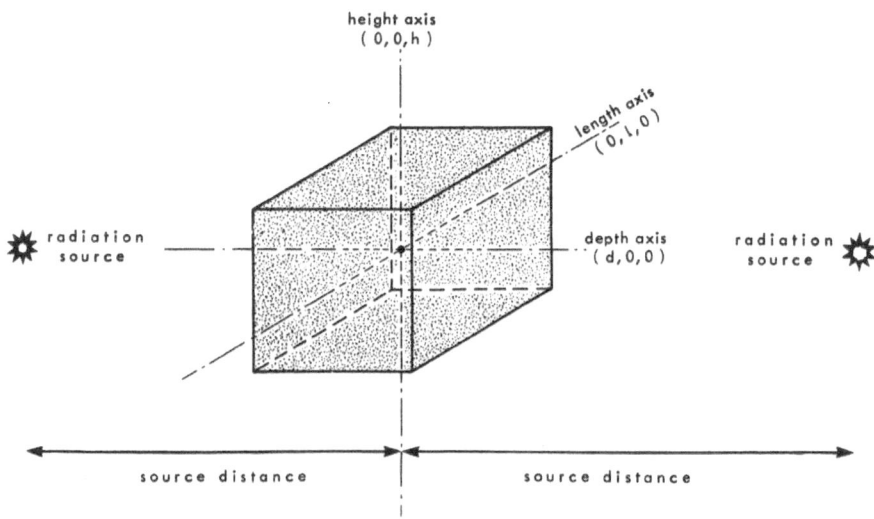

Figure 1: Irradiation arrangement for studies on dose distributions in various phantoms.

Table 2

Ratio of maximum to minimum absorbed dose along the beam axis in block-shaped acrylic plastic
phantoms of different size irradiated uni (U) and bilaterally (B) with 300 kV X rays (HVL: 3mm Cu) or
^{60}Co γ rays according to the geometry shown in Figure 1

Simulated animal	phantom height	dimensions (mm) depth (in beam direction)	length	300 kV X rays distance 0.5 m U	B	distance 1 m U	B	distance 1.5 m U	B	^{60}Co γ rays distance 0.5 m U	B	distance 1.5 m U	B
mouse	20	25	67	1.50	1.02*	1.42	1.01*	1.41	1.02*	1.24	1.00	1.13	1.01*
rat	40	40	150	1.85	1.03*	1.72	1.04*	1.64	1.04*	1.39	1.00	1.23	1.01*
rat	50	50	150	2.06	1.03*	1.88	1.04*	1.84	1.03*	1.51	1.06	1.31	1.01*
monkey	105	118	364	5.03	1.05**	4.20	1.01**	4.01	1.01**	–	–	1.95	1.00
dog	200	210	738	–	· –	–	–	9.58	1.20**	–	–	3.3i	1.07**

* dose in centre of phantom higher than at entrance planes for bilateral irradiation.

** dose in centre of phantom lower than at entrance planes for bilateral irradiation.

The uncertainty in the relative absorbed dose values is estimated to be 2 per cent.

As expected the penetration characteristics of ^{60}Co γ rays are superior to that of 300kV X rays. To obtain a homogeneous dose distribution ($D_{max}/D_{min} < 1.10$, see section 3) bilateral irradiation is required. For bilateral irradiation with the exception of the dog phantom the differences between the depth-dose distributions of the two types of radiation are small. For irradiation of the dog phantom with 300kV X rays even bilateral irradiation is not sufficient to obtain a uniform depth dose distribution. In Table 3, the maximum to minimum absorbed doses for cubes of different size irradiated unilaterally with ^{137}Cs and ^{60}Co γ rays and 4MV X rays are given. Even for 4MV X rays, unilateral irradiation of the smallest cube results in a nonuniform dose distribution.

Table 3

Ratio of maximum to minimum absorbed dose for cubes of different size irradiated unilaterally with ^{137}Cs γ rays, ^{60}Co γ rays and 4MV X rays (after ICRU, 1979) according to the geometry shown in Figure 1

D_{max}/D_{min} on the central beam axis

type of radiation cube side (mm)	^{137}Cs γ rays distance 0.5 m	distance 1.5 m	^{60}Co γ rays distance 0.5 m	distance 1.5 m	4MV X rays distance 0.5 m	distance 1.5 m
40	1.39	1.25	1.35	1.21	1.28	1.16
60	1.63	1.39	1.56	1.33	1.49	1.27
80	1.93	1.56	1.81	1.46	1.70	1.38
100	2.31	1.77	2.11	1.62	1.95	1.49
120	2.76	2.00	2.46	1.78	2.25	1.63
150	3.60	2.10	3.09	2.06	2.77	1.85
200	5.63	3.27	4.49	2.61	3.96	2.30

In Figure 2, the central depth dose distribution is given with reference to the central dose for bilateral irradiation at 1.5 m distance. The depth dose distribution for the smallest phantom is uniform for both types of radiation. For the largest phantom, the homogeneity of the dose distribution for ^{60}Co γ rays is much better than for 300kV X rays (where the dose varies about 20 per cent) owing to the smaller attenuation of ^{60}Co γ rays. The depth dose variation in the phantom with 210 mm depth of smaller height irradiated with 300kV X rays shows an even larger variation (up to about 35 per cent). This has to be attributed to a smaller dose contribution of scattered radiation compared

12

to the phantom of 200 mm height.

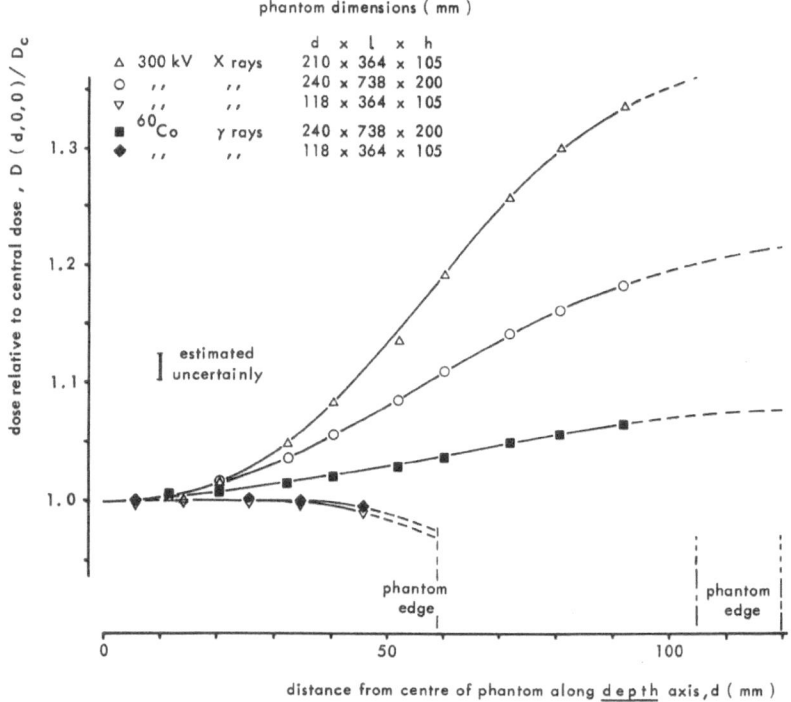

Figure 2: Relative central-axis depth dose distributions in various acrylic plastic block-shaped phantoms irradiated bilaterally at 1.5 m from the source according to the arrangement shown in Figure 1.

Dose variation along the height and length axes of a phantom (see, Figures 3 and 4) is related to a decrease in the contribution of scattered radiation "near" the edge of the phantom i.e., lack of side scatter. In addition, a dose decrease has to be expected owing to the increasing distance to the source (inverse square law attenuation) and a greater attenuation (the radiation does not enter perpendicular thus having a longer path length with increasing distance from the centre). For 300kV X rays, dependent on phantom heigth or length, dose variations in excess of 30 per cent are found. For ^{60}Co γ rays the dose variations are smaller (about 15 per cent at maximum for the largest phantom) owing to a smaller contribution of scattered radiation.

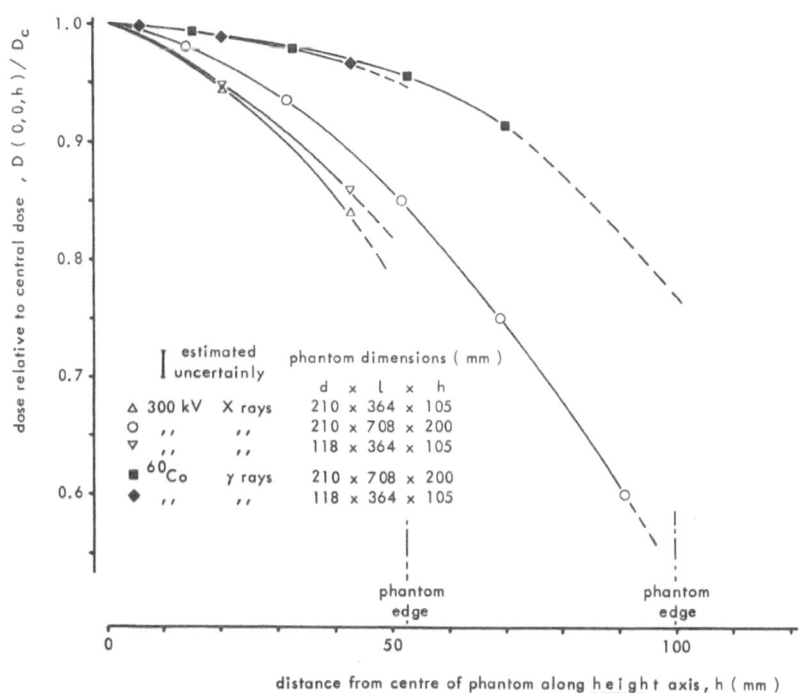

Figure 3: Relative central-axis height-dose distributions in various acrylic plastic block-shaped phantoms irradiated bilaterally at 1.5 m from the source according to the arrangement shown in Figure 1.

It is concluded that the attenuation and scattering characteristics of ^{60}Co γ rays are advantageous compared to that of 300kV X rays for obtaining a homogeneous total body irradiation of larger phantoms (animals). In general a more homogeneous dose distribution can be obtained with radiation of higher energy, provided that sufficient build-up material is used.

14

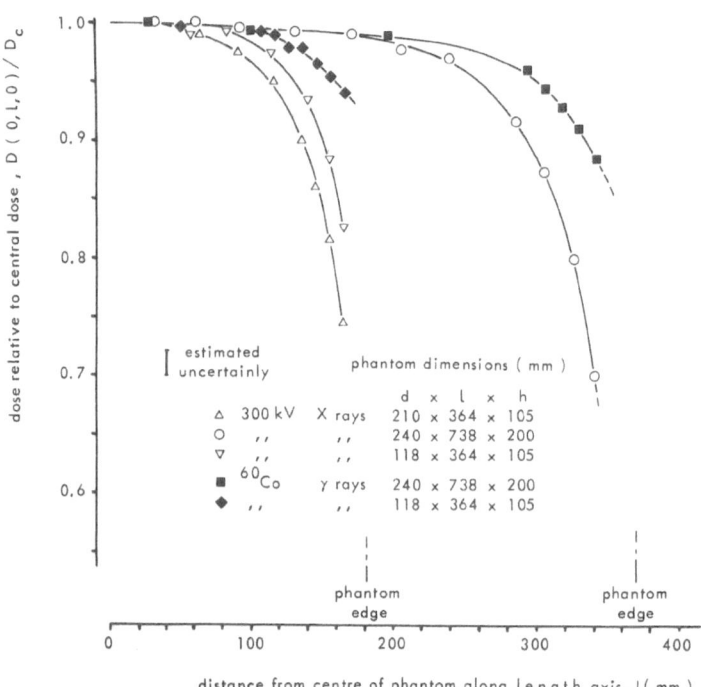

Figure 4: Relative central-axis length-dose distributions in various acrylic plastic block-shaped phantoms irradiated bilaterally at 1.5 m from the source according to the arrangement shown in Figure 1.

6.2. Phantoms of different shape

The shape of an object can influence the dose distribution appreciably. This is illustrated in Figure 5 by the dose distributions (normalized to the central dose) in the central length plane of cylindrical and block shaped phantoms of similar size irradiated bilaterally with 300kV X rays and ^{60}Co γ rays. In the block shaped phantoms, with increasing lateral distance to the centre a dose decrease is observed owing to a decreasing dose contribution (dependent on phantom size) from scattered radiation.

For the cylindrical phantoms with increasing lateral distance a dose increase can be expected due to the smaller attenuation since less material has to be traversed with increasing distance to the centre. This increase will be partly compensated for by the dose decrease due to lack of side scatter. The net result of these two counteracting processes is a larger dose increase with lateral distance for ^{60}Co γ rays than for 300kV X rays in a cylindrical phantom of the same dimensions. The results indicate that the lateral dose variations can be reduced by changing the shape of the phantom in between a block shape and a cylindrical geometry. An improvement in the depth dose distribution, however, can only be obtained by employing radiation with better penetration characteristics i.e. higher energy photons.

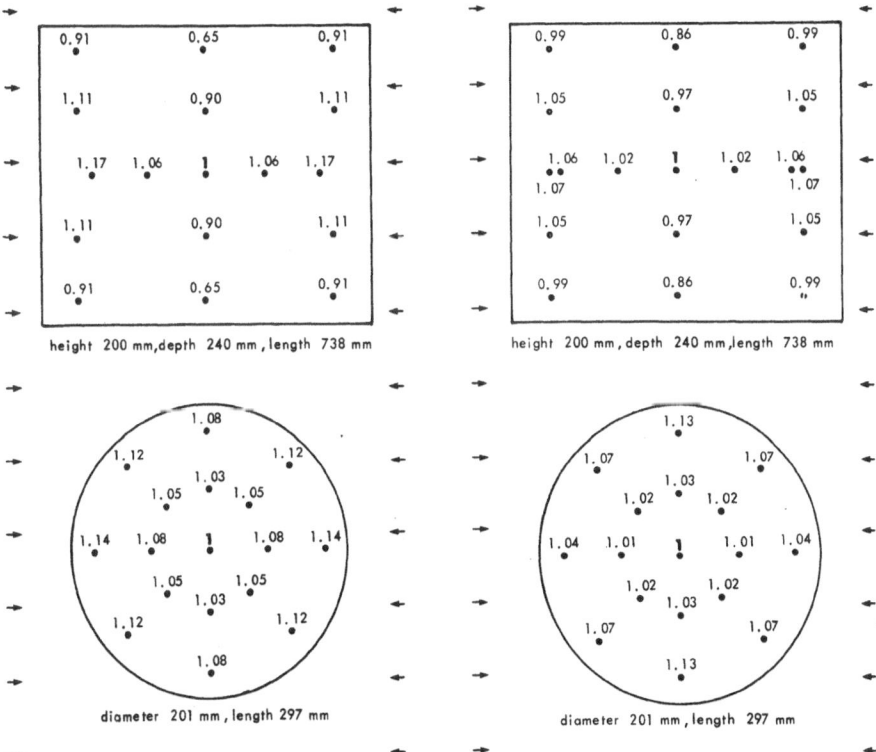

Figure 5: Relative dose in the central length plane of block-shaped and cylindrical dog phantoms irradiated bilaterally at 1.5 m from the source with 300kV X rays (left panel) and ^{60}Co γ rays (right panel) according to the arrangement shown in Figure 1.

16

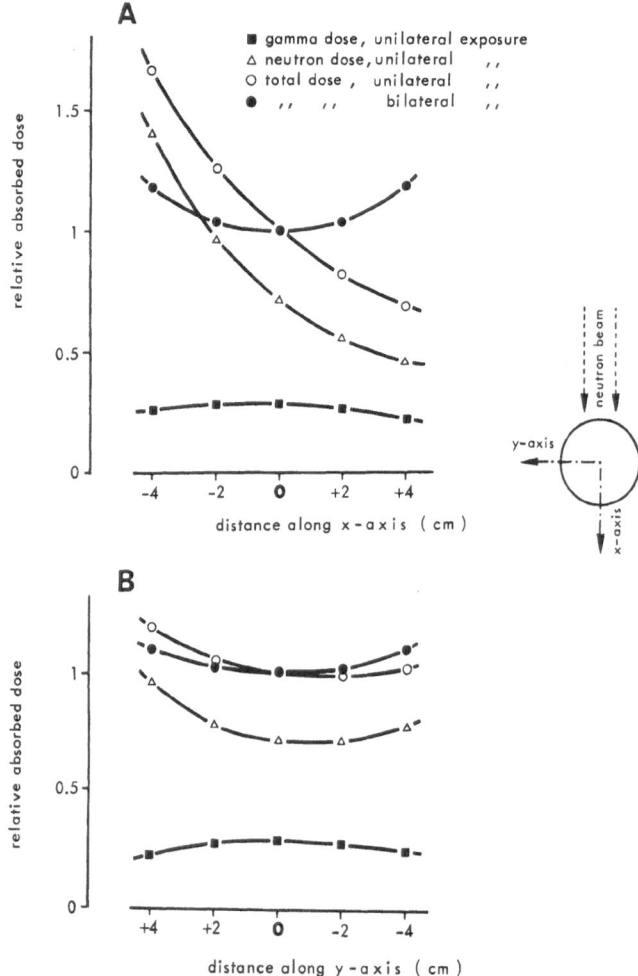

Figure 6: Dose distribution in the central length plane of a cylindrical tissue-equivalent phantom (diameter 12 cm) irradiated with fission neutrons with a mean energy of about 1 MeV (Broerse et al., 1978).

In Figure 6, the dose distribution in the central length plane of a cylindrical phantom is shown for irradiation with fission neutrons with a mean energy of about 1 MeV (Broerse et al., 1978). The phantom consists of a cylinder with an inner diameter of 12 cm filled with tissue-equivalent liquid. For neutron irradiations it is important to determine separately the neutron and photon absorbed dose components, since their relative biological effectiveness can differ considerably. This is generally achieved by a twin detector technique (see, e.g. ICRU, 1977). Bilateral irradiation is required to obtain a more homogeneous dose distribution along the central depth axis. For irradiation with neutrons, similar to the situation for photon exposures, the dose distribution in an object is determined by the scattering and attenuation characteristics of the primary radiation which are dependent on neutron energy (i.e., a reduced attenuation and scattering with increasing energy).

7. Dose distributions in inhomogeneous phantoms

The presence of body cavities, air spaces (e.g., lungs), bone and fat (particularly for fast neutrons) changes the distribution of absorbed dose in the specimen. The dosimetry problems at interfaces of materials of different composition have already been indicated in section 5. Due to their lower density the lungs are an important cause for dose inhomogeneity in whole body irradiations.

Broerse et al. (1975) measured the depth dose distributions for irradiation with d+T neutrons in a homogeneous water phantom and for the inhomogeneous situation where lung shaped containers filled with lung equivalent material were immersed in the phantom. For the total absorbed dose, at depths smaller than the entrance surface of the lungs, a steeper dose decrease is observed for the inhomogeneous phantom compared to the homogeneous situation due to a reduction in the contribution from scattered radiation in presence of the lungs. The depth dose curve inside the lungs has a reduced slope compared to the slope in water owing to the lower density of the lungs. The complex balance between differences in attenuation and scattering caused by the presence of lungs will determine the net effect. For d+T neutrons the average total dose in the lungs is increased compared to that in the equivalent volume in the homogeneous phantom. The influence of the presence of lungs on the dose distributions for the photon component show similarities with the situation for the total absorbed dose, however, the situation is somewhat different due to the production of photons by neutron interactions in the object.

Marinello et al. (1982) determined lung correction factors for whole body irradiations with ^{60}Co γ rays. They measured doses inside block-shaped volumes of lung equivalent material enclosed in block-shaped volumes of tissue-equivalent material (polystyrene) and compared the values with measurements at the same positions in a homogeneous polystyrene phantom of the same size. The lung correction factor (i.e., the ratio of the dose in the centre of the lung to the dose at the same position in the homogeneous phantom) was measured to be equal to 1.05, 1.14 and 1.24 for lung thicknesses of 5, 12 and 18 cm, respectively. It was further concluded that, for ^{60}Co γ rays the influence of side scatter and lung height and width are of minor importance and that the main effect is related to the dimensions in the beam direction i.e., lung thickness and thickness of overlaying tissue.

8. Tissue-air ratio

Under certain conditions it may not be possible to determine absorbed dose (e.g., at interfaces of different materials). In some investigations (e.g., retrospective studies) information on the absorbed dose (distribution) in the biological object is not available. Many measurement devices are designed and calibrated for measurements under free-in-air conditions and their use inside an object can give rise to unexpected difficulties and larger uncertainties. Therefore, it can be convenient to specify the midline kerma in air under receptor-free conditions as a reference quantity (ICRU, 1979). For photon irradiations the midline exposure may be used instead of midline kerma. For derivation of the absorbed dose (distribution) in an object it is essential that, in addition to midline kerma in air, information is provided on the irradiation source and geometry and the location, dimensions and composition of the irradiated object.

The tissue air ratio (TAR) is defined as the ratio of the absorbed dose (rate) at a given point in a phantom to the absorbed dose (rate) at the same point in free space, but at the centre of a small amount of phantom material just large enough to provide secondary charged particle equilibrium at the point of measurement (ICRU, 1979). TAR can be used to convert kerma at the midline position into central absorbed dose. In Table 4, TAR values for the central positions of various phantoms are given for irradiations with 300kV X rays and ^{60}Co γ rays. It is concluded from the table that the TAR for the central phantom positions are dependent on type of radiation, phantom dimensions, source to centre of phantom distance and shape of the phantom.

Table 4

Tissue-air ratio for the centre positions of various block shaped acrylic plastic and some cylindrical phantoms irradiated with 300 kV X rays and ^{60}Co γ rays according to an arrangement as shown in Figure 1

| simulated animal | phantom dimension (mm) | | | 300 kV X rays | | ^{60}Co γ rays | |
	height	depth (in beam direction)	length	distance 0.5 m	distance 1.5 m	distance 0.5 m	distance 1.5 m
mouse	20	25	67	1.00	1.00	0.96	0.98
rat	40	40	150	1.03	1.02	0.95	0.97
rat	50	50	150	1.04	1.03	0.94	0.96
monkey	105	118	364	1.01	0.96	-	0.88
dog	215	240	738	-	0.83	-	0.74
	diameter (mm)		length (mm)				
monkey	125		297	0.90	0.86	-	0.89
dog	201		297	-	0.74	-	0.80

9. Methods to improve the dose distribution

It has been demonstrated (see, section 6) that radiation scattering has a large effect on the dose variation in a (biological) object. For small animals (e.g., rats and mice) usually a number of these are irradiated simultaneously and the effect of side scattering of adjacent animals has to be taken into account. Back and side scatter material can be used to improve the dose distribution. From Figures 2, 3 and 4, by comparing the dose distributions in the phantoms of smaller size with those inside phantoms of larger dimensions, it can be derived that the addition of scatter material will improve the dose distribution. From Figure 5 it is concluded that the lateral dose distribution inside an object can be improved by the addition of bolus material so that the shape of the object will be of a suitable geometry (intermediate between a cylindrical and a block shape depending on type of radiation). The use of higher energy photons or neutrons will generally improve the depth dose distribution since their penetration characteristics are better (smaller attenuation and less scatter).

Multilateral irradiation will improve the absorbed dose distribution inside objects (see, e.g., Figures 5 and 6). The presence of lungs will result in general in an increased absorbed dose in these organs owing to their lower density (see, section 7). This can partly be compensated for by the addition of a layer of bolus material or shielding.

10. Example of the biological consequences of an inhomogeneous dose distribution

A comparison is made between the central doses required to produce the same biological effect in inhomogeneous and homogeneous irradiations of a block-shaped uniform cell distribution.

Given a homogeneous distribution of cells in a block with thickness,

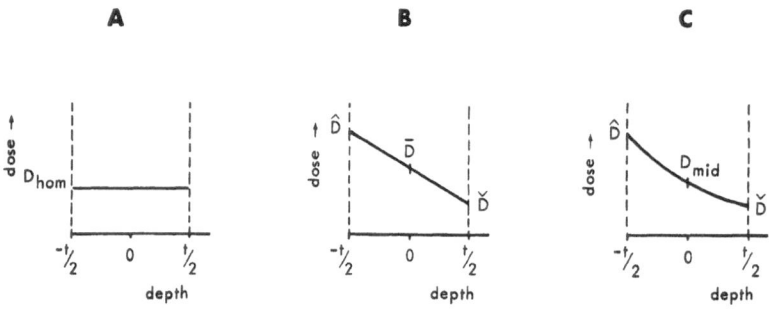

Figure 7: Schematic depth dose distributions inside a block-shaped object of thickness, t.
Panel A: Homogeneous dose distribution.
Panel B: Linear dose distribution as a function of depth. Indicated are: maximum (entrance) dose, $\hat{D}$, the mean (central) dose, $\bar{D}$, and the minimum (exit) dose, $\check{D}$.
Panel C: Exponential depth dose curve, where D_{mid} is the dose at the central position of the phantom.

t. In case of a homogeneous irradiation (see, Figure 7A) the dose is constant over the depth in the object, D_{hom}. For the inhomogeneous irradiation (see, Figure 7B) it is assumed that the dose varies linearly with depth between the maximum dose, $\hat{D}$ and the minimum dose, $\check{D}$ and $\bar{D}$ is the mean as well as the central dose. In both ways of irradiation it is assumed further that the dose along the height and length axes is constant. The fraction of surviving cells $S(D)$ at a dose D is given by the relation:

$$S(D) = e^{-\alpha D} \tag{1}$$

For the homogeneous irradiation the fraction of surviving cells is represented by:

$$S_{hom}(D_{hom}) = e^{-\alpha D_{hom}} \tag{2}$$

For the inhomogeneous irradiation, taking $\hat{D}-\check{D}$ as a measure for the inhomogeneity, follows:

$$S_{inhom,lin}(\bar{D},\hat{D}-\check{D}) = \frac{1}{t}\int_{-t/2}^{t/2} e^{-\alpha\left[\bar{D} - \frac{(\hat{D}-\check{D})}{t}x\right]} dx$$

$$= \frac{e^{-\alpha\bar{D}}\sinh \tfrac{1}{2}\alpha(\hat{D}-\check{D})}{\tfrac{1}{2}\alpha(\hat{D}-\check{D})} \tag{3}$$

To obtain an equal effect for the different ways of irradiation $S_{hom}(D_{hom})$ should be equal to $S_{inhom,lin}(\bar{D},\hat{D}-\check{D})$ and consequently the following relation exists for the doses in the two situations:

$$\alpha D_{hom} = \alpha\bar{D} - \ln\frac{\sinh \tfrac{1}{2}\alpha(\hat{D}-\check{D})}{\tfrac{1}{2}\alpha(\hat{D}-\check{D})} \tag{4}$$

A more realistic dose distribution as a function of depth is represented by exponential attenuation (see, Figure 7C), where $\hat{D}$ and $\check{D}$ are the entrance and exit doses, respectively, and D_{mid} the central dose. For the exponential dose decrease with depth x in the block the following relation is valid:

$$D(x) = D_{mid} \ e^{- \frac{x}{t} \ln(\hat{D}/\check{D})} \qquad\qquad -t/2 \ll x \ll t/2 \qquad (5)$$

The fraction of surviving cells as a function of the central dose, D_{mid} and the inhomogeneity of the dose, $\hat{D}/\check{D}$, can be formulated as:

$$S_{inhom,exp} = \frac{1}{t} \int_{-t/2}^{t/2} e^{-\alpha D_{mid} \ e^{- \frac{x}{t} \ln(\hat{D}/\check{D})}} \ dx \qquad (6)$$

The relation between the dose in a homogeneous irradiation, D_{hom} and the central dose, D_{mid} (in case of an exponential dose decrease with depth) to obtain the same amount of cell survival can be derived from:

$$\alpha D_{hom} = \alpha D_{mid} - \ln \left[\frac{1}{t} \int_{-t/2}^{t/2} e^{-\alpha D_{mid} \ (e^{- \frac{x}{t} \ln(\hat{D}/\check{D})} -1)} \ dx \right] \qquad (7)$$

Equation 7 has been solved numerically as shown in Figure 8 where αD_{hom} is plotted against αD_{mid} for various values of $\hat{D}/\check{D}$. In Table 5 the influence of the inhomogeneity of the dose distribution on the dose-effect relations is illustrated by using data of Vriesendorp and Van Bekkum (1980) on the occurrence of the bone marrow sydrome in different species. It is evident that the central dose, D_{mid}, in an inhomogeneous irradiation required to produce the same biological effect as the dose in a uniform irradiation has to be considerably higher (dependent on the degree of inhomogeneity). Consequently, the use of D_{mid} without knowledge of the dose and cellular distribution can lead to a severe underestimation of the biological effect in homogeneous irradiations.

Table 5

Example of the influence of an inhomogeneous dose distribution (characterized by D_{mid} and $\hat{D}/\check{D}$) on $LD_{50/30}$ in several animals based on data of Vriesendorp and Van Bekkum (1980). It is assumed that the animals are block shaped, the haemopoietic stem cells are distributed uniform throughout the block, the dose decreases exponentially as a function of depth and cell survival is according to: $lnS = -\alpha D$

| species $\hat{D}/\check{D}$ | $S(LD_{50/30})$ – | $LD_{50/30}$ (Gy) – | αD_{hom} at $LD_{50/30}$ – | \multicolumn{11}{c}{$(LD_{50/30})_{mid}$ (Gy)} |
				1.05	1.10	1.30	1.50	1.70	2.00	2.50	3.00	4.00	5.00	8.00
mouse	10^{-5}	7.0	11.5	7.0	7.03	7.2	7.5	7.7	8.2	8.9	9.6	10.8	11.9	14.7
rat	3.10^{-5}	6.75	10.4	6.75	6.77	6.9	7.2	7.4	7.8	8.5	9.1	10.3	11.3	13.8
monkey	10^{-4}	5.25	9.2	5.25	5.27	5.4	5.5	5.7	6.0	6.5	7.0	7.8	8.5	10.4
dog	6.10^{-4}	3.7	7.4	3.7	3.71	3.8	3.9	4.0	4.1	4.4	4.7	5.3	5.7	7.0

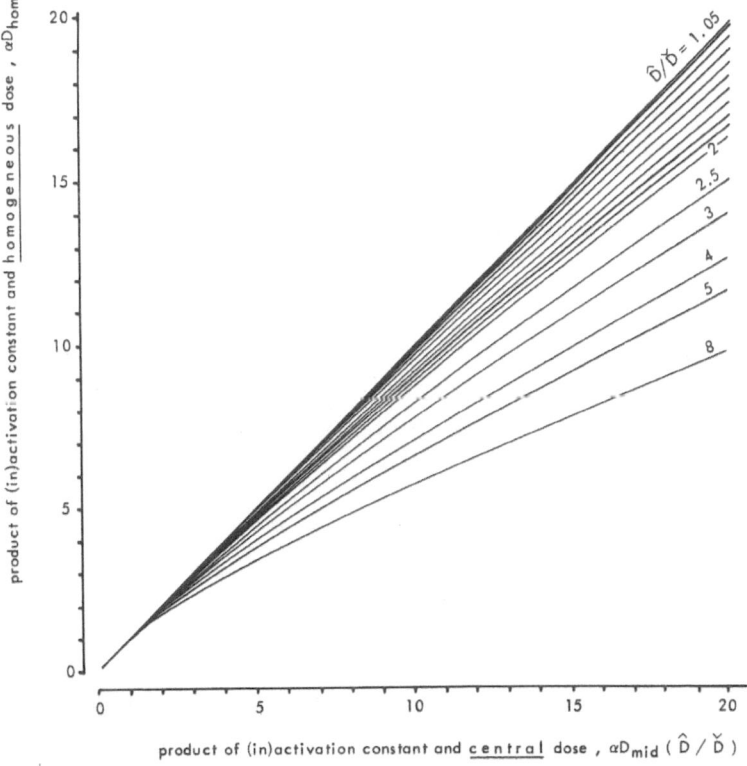

Figure 8: Relation between the doses required to produce the same biological effect (in case of only a linear dose term, α) for homogeneous and inhomogeneous irradiation of a block-shaped uniform distribution of biological entities (e.g., cells). The homogeneous dose is specified by D_{hom}. The inhomogeneous exponential dose distribution as function of depth is characterized by the central dose, D_{mid} and the ratio of maximum to minimum absorbed dose, $\hat{D}/\check{D}$ (see, Figure 7c). The doses along height and length axes of the object are assumed to be constant.

24

11. Summary and conclusions

The dosimetry procedures for irradiation of biological objects are shown schematically in Figure 9. Some dosimetric aspects have been dicussed in previous sections, others will be briefly reviewed below.

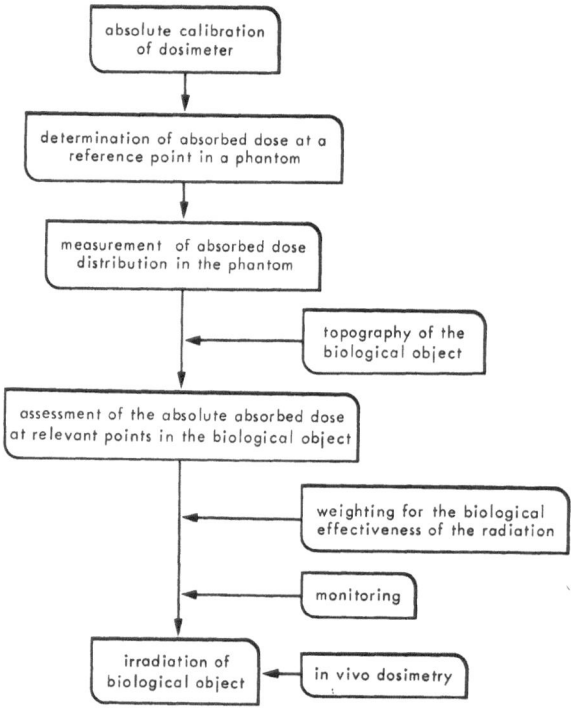

Figure 9: Schematic representation of dosimetry procedures for irradiation of a biological object.

Most dosimeters do not provide a direct measure of absorbed dose but require calibration in a known radiation field. For ionization chambers it is recommended that a regular calibration of these devices is performed at or is traceable to a standards laboratory, at least once a year. At present the quantity used for photon calibration at the standardization institutes is the exposure. Consequently, the conversion of exposure to absorbed dose is left to the user. For neutrons, a calibration of dosimeters in a standard neutron field is not yet possible, but a calibration in a photon field can be used as a basis for neutron dosimetry. Preferably the calibration of a dosimeter should be performed in a radiation field resembling as closely as possible that actually employed for the radiobiological experiments. To ascertain the stability of the dosimetry systems during the time intervals between calibrations it is essential to have a control system. Usually for this purpose check sources in a fixed arrangement are employed.

The absolute determination of absorbed dose at a reference point inside a homogeneous medium (phantom) is an essential step in the procedures followed for specification of absorbed dose. In radiotherapy commonly acrylic plastic cubes (with outside dimensions of about 30cm) filled with water are used as volumes of tissue-substitute material, to provide full scatter conditions for the beams investigated. The reference points for dosimetry are generally located on the central beam axis at 5 or 10 cm depth. This information is important for exchange of biomedical data between different centres and for a comparison and interpretation of the effectiveness of different types of radiation for inducing biological effects.

Subsequent to the determination of the absolute dose at a reference point, information should be obtained about the relative absorbed dose distribution in a reference phantom (see, section 6). The dose distribution inside a phantom for whole body irradiation is determined by the complex (partly balancing) attenuation and scatter characteristics of the primary radiation and is dependent on phantom size and shape, distance to the source, uni- or bilateral exposure and type of irradiation. The uniformity of the dose distribution can be improved in general by using higher primary particle energies, multilateral exposure and addition of bolus and scatter material (see, section 9). Experimental dose determinations require considerable beam production and measurement time, therefore, systems for computation of the dose pattern have been developed.

To provide information on the dose distribution in the biological system actually irradiated, often realistic phantoms are used. These phantoms are generally constructed in such a way that the dimensions, shape and chemical composition are similar to the object to be irradiated. The requirements for dose specification and dose delivery are indicated in section 3. The presence of the lungs is commonly a major cause for dose inhomogeneity (see, section 7), but dose variations will also occur at interfaces of materials of different atomic composition (see, section 5). This latter aspect requires knowledge about the topography of the object and the location of critical biological targets. The biological consequences of inhomogeneous dose distributions are illustrated by a simple model (see section 10).

For conventional X-ray machines and isotopic sources, monitoring makes it possible to detect defaults in electrical and mechanical systems involved such as source position errors, jammed shutters and improper or malplaced filters. Continuous monitoring of the beam intensity is essential when accelerators are used. These complex machines and associated beam steering systems cannot be relied upon to operate over relatively long time periods at an output sufficiently constant for biomedical purposes. The relationship between monitor response and absorbed dose at a reference point in a phantom should be determined. Changes in field size or scattering material can influence this relation as well as the dose distribution pattern.

For the actual irradiation of a biological object the information on radation quality has to be taken into account as a weighting factor for the biological effectiveness of the radiation. Information on radiation quality can be given by a specification of microdosimetric quantities, but also by information on the energy spectrum of the radiation. For X rays the half value layer (HVL) thickness can be used as an indication for radiation quality.

In vivo dosimetry provides the possibility of checking the procedures to convert absorbed doses in reference phantoms to absorbed doses in the complex biological objects actually irradiated. In addition, in vivo dosimeters can be used for the verification of treatment planning and control procedures. Dosimeters suitable for attachment to skin or introduction in body cavities include TLD and semiconductor detectors.

Acknowledgements

The skilled technical assistance of Messrs A.C. Engels, C.J. Bouts and N.J.P. de Wit in the measurements is gratefully acknowledged. The authors express their gratitude to Mrs. F.G. Pluimers for typing the manuscript and Mr. J.Ph. de Kler for preparing the figures.

References

Broerse, J.J., Barendsen, G.W. and Kersen, G.R. van, 1968. Survival of cultured human cells after irradiation with neutrons of different energies in hypoxic and oxygenated conditions. Int.J.Radiat.Biol., 13, 559-572.

Broerse, J.J., Broers-Challiss, J.E. and Mijnheer, B.J., 1975. Depth dose measurements of d-T neutrons for radiotherapy applications. Strahlentherapy, 149, 585-596.

Broerse, J.J., and Mijnheer, B.J., 1982. Accuracy and precision of absorbed dose measurements for neutron therapy. Int.J.Rad.Oncology Biol.Phys., 8, 2049-2056.

Fricke, F.S. and Hart, E.J., 1966. Chemical dosimetry. In: Radiation Dosimetry vol. II (eds. Attix, F.II. and Roesch, W.C.), pp. 167-239, Academic Press, New York.

Gunn, S.R., 1976. Radiometric calorimetry: A review. Nucl.Inst.Meth., 135, 251-265.

ICRU, 1969. Report 14. Radiation dosimetry: X rays and gamma rays with maximum photon energies between 0.6 and 50 MeV. ICRU, Washington.

ICRU, 1977. Report 26. Neutron dosimetry for biology and medicine. ICRU, Washington.

ICRU, 1979. Report 30. Quantitative concepts and dosimetry in radiobiology. ICRU, Washington.

ICRU, 1980. Report 33. Radiation quantities and units. ICRU, Washington.

Marinello, G., Barrie, A.M., Bourgeois, J.P. le, 1982. Measurements and calculation of lung dose in total body irradiations performed with ^{60}Co. J.Eur.Radiother., 3, 174-182.

Maughan, R.L., Slabbert, J.P. and Roper, M.J., 1983. Use of the modified Fricke solution (FBX) for neutron dosimetry. In: Proc. seventh int. congress of radiation research (eds. Broerse, J.J., Barendsen, G.W., Kal, H.B. and Kogel, A.J. van der) session E2-27.

Rossi, H.H., 1968. Microscopic energy distribution in irradiated matter. In: Radiation Dosimetry. Vol. I (eds. Attix, F.H. and Roesch, W.C.) pp. 43-92. Academic Press, New York.

Sinclair, W.K., 1969. Radiobiological dosimetry. In: Radiation Dosimetry, Vol. III (eds. Attix, F.H. and Tochilin, E.) pp. 627-676. Academic Press, New York.

Vriesendorp, H.M. and Bekkum, D.W. van, 1980. Role of total body irradiation in conditioning for bone marrow transplantation. In: Immuno-biology of bone marrow transplantation (eds. Thierfelder, S., Rodt, H. and Kolb, H.J.) pp. 349-364, Springer Verlag, Berlin.

Zoetelief, J. 1981. Dosimetry and biological effects of fast neutrons. Thesis, Amsterdam.

Dose and Cell-Survival Calculations in Anthropomorphic Phantoms

Dean C. Kaul[1] and William H. Scott[2]

Science Applications, Inc., [1]1701 E. Woodfield Rd., Suite 819, Schaumburg, Illinois 60195, [2]1200 Prospect St. (P.O. Box 2351), La Jolla, California 92038, USA.

Science Applications, Inc. (SAI) has performed calculations of marrow dose and marrow cell survival in anthropomorphic phantoms for the Defense Nuclear Agency (1) and for the Bundeswehr (2,3). That work has recently been expanded to include dose calculations for all organs in a family of Japanese anthropomorphic phantoms. The latter effort is in support of the dose re-analysis for the A-bomb survivors, now on-going (4).

Recently, SAI has calculated a number of dose and related parameters in an anthropomorphic phantom standing erect in a radiation field typical of a low yield tactical nuclear weapon. A view of the internal detail (skeleton and lung) of the phantom is shown in Figure 1. The phantom is representative of adult western man as modeled by Cristy (5). The radiation field is characterized as shown in Figure 2. The high neutron-to-gamma ray dose ratio is typical of a low yield weapon.

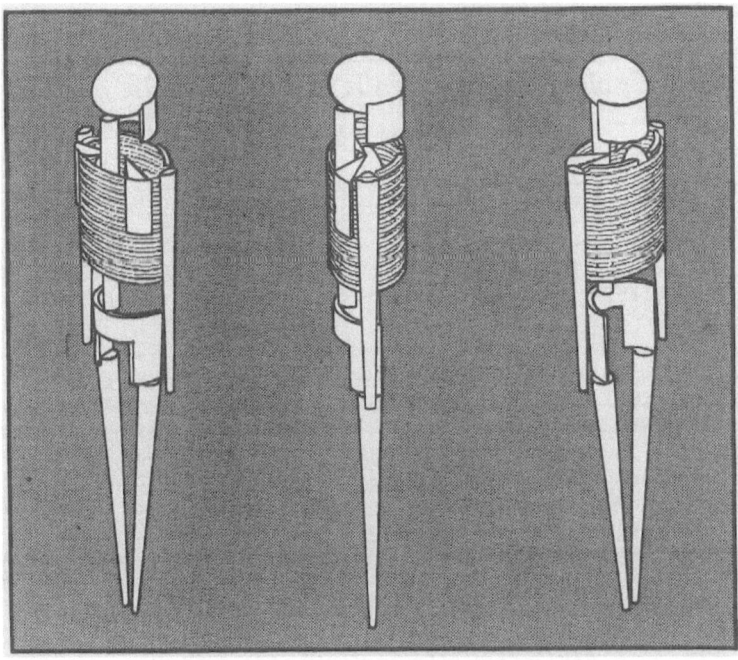

Figure 1. Man phantom models interior detail skeleton and lungs.

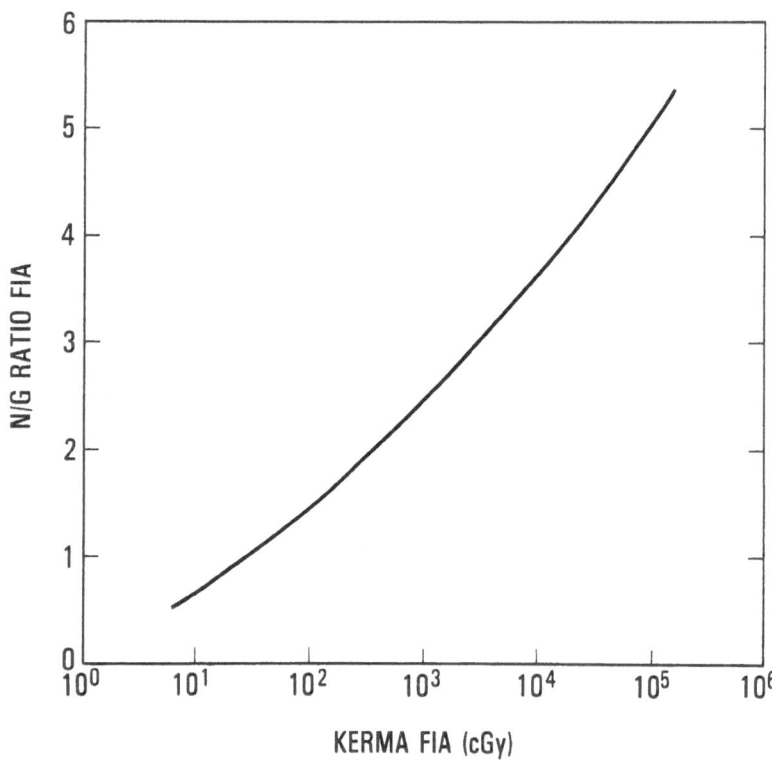

Figure 2. Tactical Free Field Radiation. Neutron/gamma (N/G) ratio relative to Kerma as measured free-in-air (FIA).

Calculations of dose and other quantities within the phantom situated in the radiation field are accomplished by SAI using the Vehicle Code System (VCS) Code (6). This code permits the linear coupling of angular fluences, calculated using a two-dimensional discrete ordinates transport code, with the adjoint angular fluence, calculated using a three-dimensional Monte Carlo transport code. This process is depicted in Figure 3. The free-field environment is calculated in two dimensions, while the transport within the phantom is calculated in the adjoint mode in three dimensions. The product of the forward-adjoint coupling procedure is the energy-differential fluence within any dosimetric region of interest within the phantom.

$$\phi(E') = \int_E \int_\Omega \phi(E,\Omega) * \phi'(E,\Omega \to E') \ d\Omega dE$$

where ϕ is the incident fluence, differential in energy (E) and angle (Ω) and ϕ' is the adjoint fluence, differential in energy (E) and angle (Ω), relative to energy (E'), and

$$D_{i,j,k} = \int_{E'} K_i dE' \int \int_\Omega \phi(E,\Omega) * \phi'(E,\Omega \rightarrow E') d\Omega dE$$

where D is the kerma (K) weighted fluence for the ith organ of the jth phantom in the kth posture.

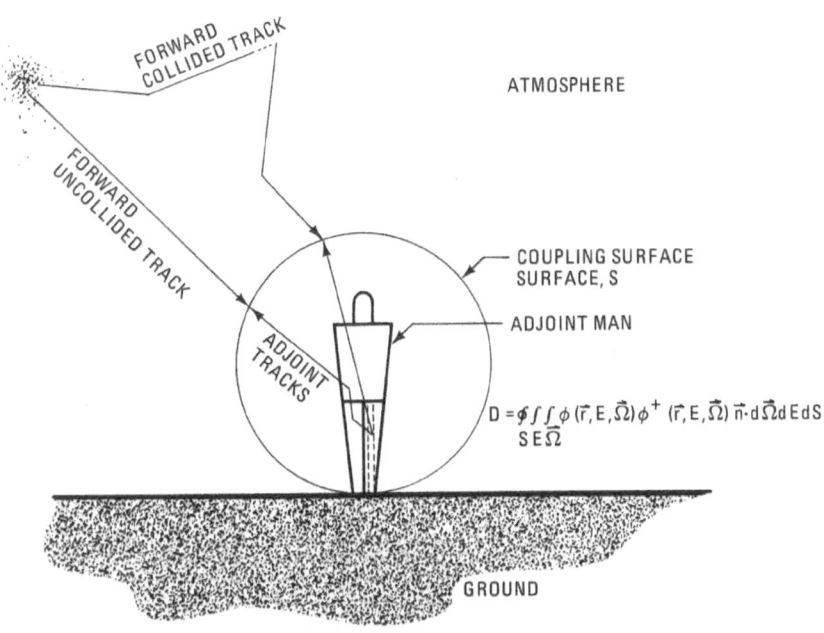

Figure 3. Illustration of forward-adjoint coupling.

SAI has calculated radiation transmission to the mid-head, mid-thorax and marrow in the radiation field from a tactical device. The results have been obtained for three different orientations of man standing erect on the ground surface. The first orientation is facing ground-zero (A-P), the second is facing normal to the ground-zero direction (side) and, finally, facing away from ground-zero (P-A). The mid-head results (Figure 4) show that the side exposure provides for consistently greater transmission than does the P-A orientation. This is because the phantom head is elliptical, having its minor axis in the lateral direction. The results for these two orientations reflect the diminishing neutron-to-gamma ray kerma ratio in the incident-free field, with the transmission increasing by approximately 30% from the highest to the lowest kerma levels (shortest to longest ranges). The results for the A-P orientation are something of an anomaly, depicting a significant decrease in the transmission at high kerma levels. This is particularly true with respect to dose from incident neutrons. At low kerma levels the gamma ray transmission is enhanced well above that for other orientations. A study of the phantom geometry gives no indication of the cause of the A-P transmission fluctuations. It may be that the problem lies in the Monte Carlo statistics. This possibility is being investigated, although the reported fractional standard deviations (FSD) for these transmission factors are between 0.05 and 0.10, usually considered an acceptable range.

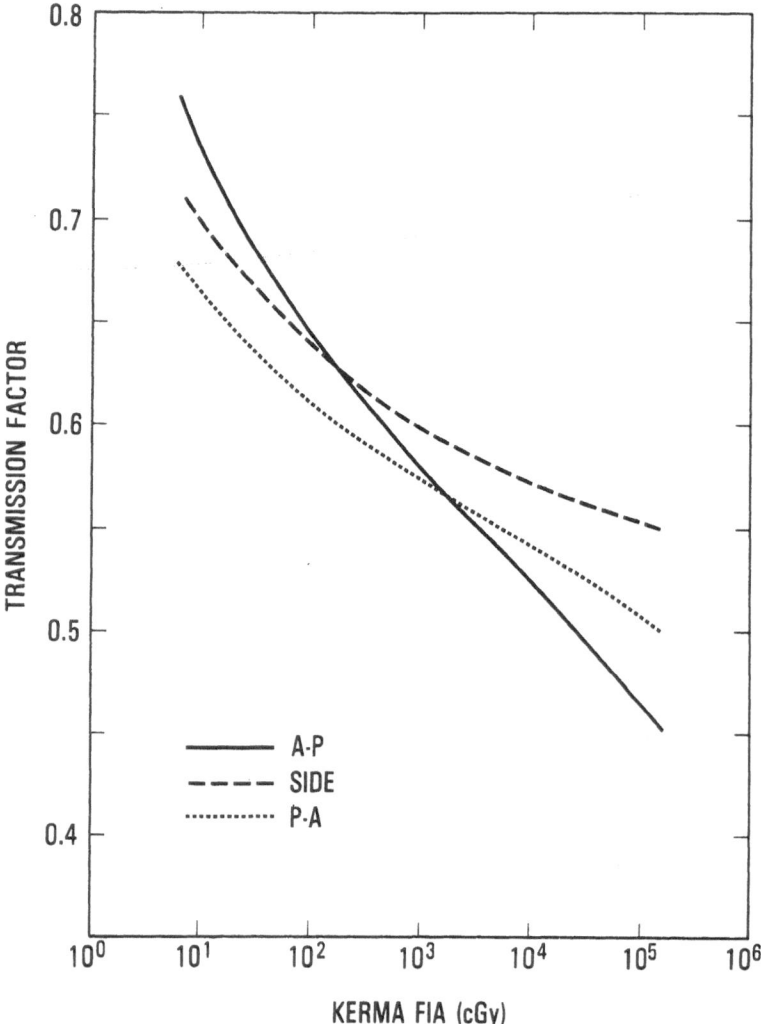

Figure 4. Dose transmission versus free-in-air kerma in the mid-head for different orientations; A-P (solid), side (dashed), P-A (dotted) lines.

The neutron-to-gamma ray dose ratios for the mid-head show a reduction from the free field values of a factor of seven at high kerma levels and a factor of four at low kerma levels. This varies somewhat with orientation. The side exposure enhances the neutron-to-gamma ray dose ratio, particularly at the high kerma levels.

The mid-thorax dose transmission is shown in Figure 5. The transmission factors for A-P and side orientation display similar behavior. The A-P transmission is greater than that from the side due to the elliptical shape of the phantom trunk. Because of the large dimensions of the trunk relative to those of the head, the transmission into the former varies even more with changes in neutron-to-gamma ray kerma ratio than does that for the latter location. In fact, the increase in transmission from the highest to lowest kerma levels is nearly a factor of two. The transmission factor of the P-A orientation appears to exhibit anomalous behavior as did that for the mid-head A-P orientation. However, in this case the phantom geometry provides some explanation for

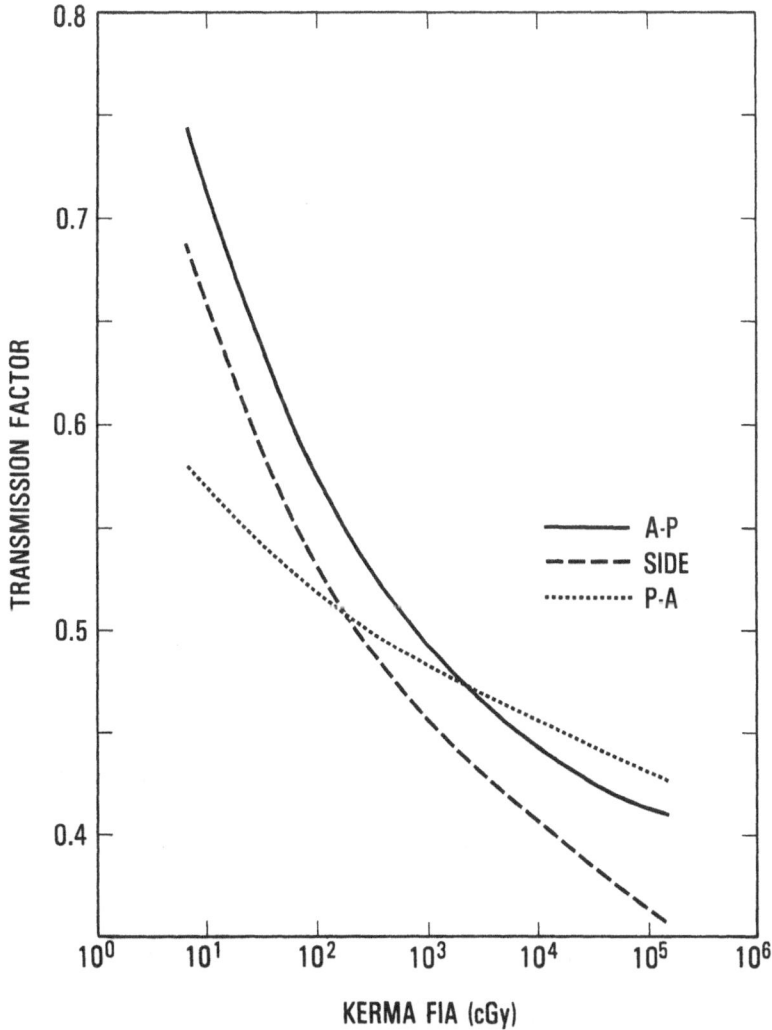

Figure 5. Dose transmission versus free-in-air kerma in the mid-thorax for different orientations; A-P (solid), side (dashed), P-A (dotted) lines.

the behavior. The neutron transmission is enhanced by virtue of the low density lung tissue which is biased toward the rear of the phantom. Thus, the overall transmission is increased at high kerma levels. On the other hand, the spine shields the mid-thorax from highly directional gamma rays. Thus, the transmission is reduced at the lowest kerma values. This explanation seems plausible. However, the FSD for these transmission factors is approximately 0.10 for gamma rays and between 0.10 and 0.20 for neutrons. Thus, statistical uncertainty could also be responsible for the P-A transmission anomaly.

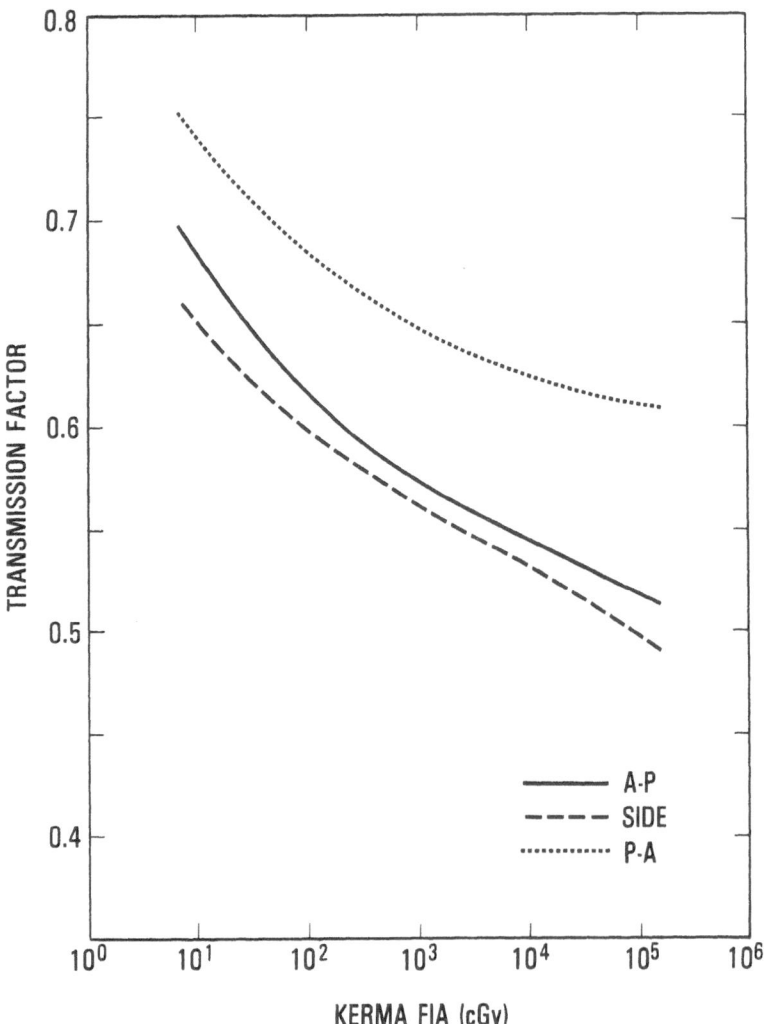

Figure 6. Dose transmission versus free-in-air kerma in the marrow for different orientations; A-P (solid), side (dashed), P-A (dotted) lines.

Transmission to the marrow (Figure 6) and neutron-to-gamma dose ratios in the marrow (Figure 7) depict similar variations across the entire kerma range for all three orientations, varying by approximately 30% from high to low kerma values. The P-A orientation is favored for neutron and, to a lesser extent, gamma ray transmission. This is because the marrow distribution is biased toward the rear of the phantom. The side exposure provides the least transmission overall. However, the angular distribution of the neutrons allows them access to the posterior

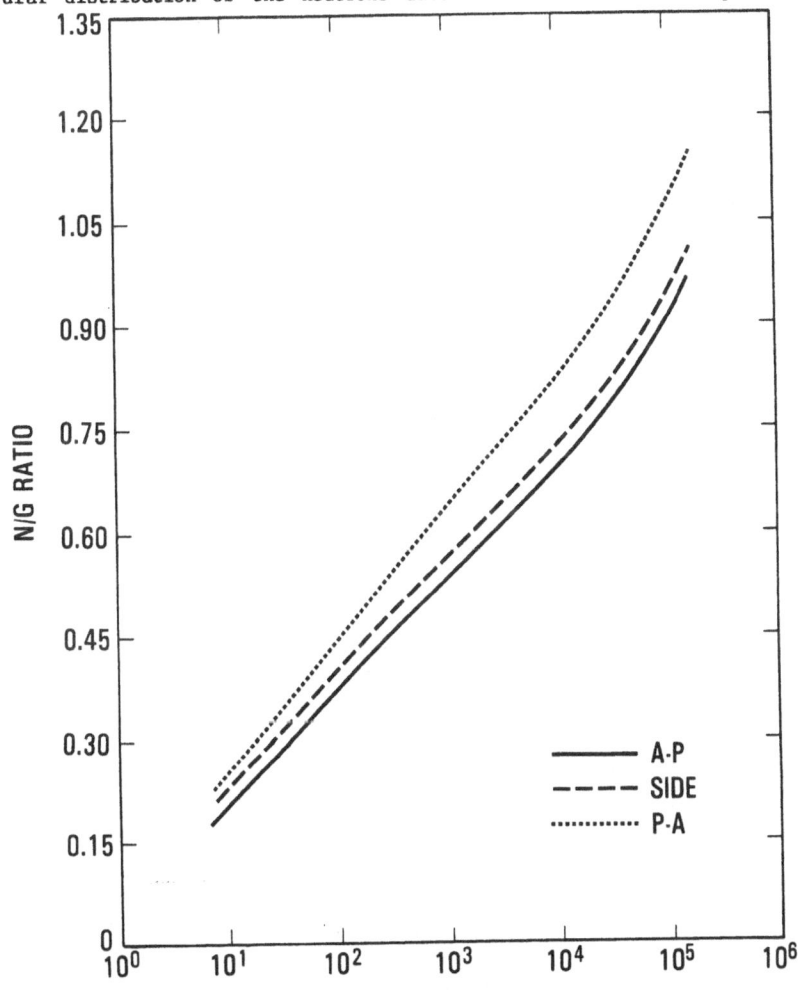

Figure 7. Marrow neutron/gamma ratio versus free-in-air kerma in the for different orientations; A-P (solid), side (dashed), P-A (dotted) lines.

marrow, even in the side orientation. Thus, the neutron-to-gamma ray dose ratio for the side orientation exceeds that for the A-P orientation. The neutron-to-gamma ray dose ratios are substantially reduced from the free-in-air values, though not as much as those for the mid-thorax location. That reduction varies from a factor of five at high kerma values to a factor of three at low kerma values. It should be noted that the above results are the average for all the marrow. Individual marrow regions are likely to exhibit significantly different results (1,2,3).

SAI has been active in the practical application of the model developed by Katz (7,8,9) for the prediction of cell survival in mixed LET radiation fields. According to Katz, the surviving fraction of oxygenated marrow cells exposed in vitro may be expressed as

$$\frac{N}{N_o} = \pi_I x \, \pi_\gamma$$

$$\pi_\gamma = 1 - (1-EXP\left[-\sum_J(1-P_J^\Sigma)D_J/D_o\right])^m$$

$$\pi_I = EXP\ (-\sum_J \sigma_o P_J D_J/L_J)$$

where π_γ is the fraction surviving radiation interaction in a manner like that of gamma rays, which bathe cells in a fluence of secondary electrons (gamma mode), and, π_I is the fraction surviving interaction of a concentration of such secondary electrons along the track of a heavy charged particle (ion mode). The local radiation is characterized by dose D, having a particular LET indicated by subscript J. The probability of cell kill (usually measured in terms of reproductive incapacitation) in the ion mode and the characteristic LET of radiation type J are given by P and L, respectively. The quantity σ_o is an empirically-derived parameter approximating the largest sensitive cross section of the particular cell type for high LET radiation (σ_o=4.2 x 10^{-7} cm^2 for marrow). The quantities D_o and m(=2.5) are similarly derived from exposure in low LET fields.

Values of the quantities (1-P)K and (σ_oP/L)K, where K is the appropriate kerma value (centigrays per unit fluence), have been calculated for neutron incidence on active marrow using the MACKSPAR code (10). In the case of photon incidence, P=0 and the parameters necessary for cell survival calculation are reduced to kerma alone.

SAI has used the Katz model to develop human mortality criteria based on cell survival. These criteria are based on those put forth by Langham (11), but could be used on any set of base data. The Langham data were assumed to refer to midline dose at mid-thorax due to Cs-137 photons incident in the midplane. This midline dose was translated into cell survival fraction by means of the phantom calculations and cell survival model described above. The results of this transformation are shown in Table 1. The LD$_{50}$ midline dose of 286 centigrays (rads) is translated into 13.17% marrow survival. This is a much more useful criterion than any dose value because, according to Bond and Robinson (12), if that percentage of marrow survives anywhere in the body, the criterion will apply. Thus, the marrow cell survival criterion may be used in partial shielding or fluence gradient situations, where average dose values are meaningless.

Table 1

Mortality Probability (%)	Midline Dose (rad(muscle))	Midplane Cs137 Photon Fluence (γ c cm^{-2})	Average Marrow Dose (rad(marrow))	Marrow Cell Survival Fraction
99	406	1.713×10^{12}	379	4.116×10^{-2}
98	392	1.654	366	4.719
95	371	1.566	346	5.783
93	362	1.528	338	6.313
90	352	1.486	329	6.960
80	329	1.388	307	8.710
70	313	1.320	292	1.018×10^{-1}
60	299	1.262	280	1.162
50	286±25(S.E.M)*	1.207±.106	267±23	$1.317^{+.356}_{-.282}$
40	273	1.152	255	1.491
30	259	1.093	242	1.703
20	243	1.026	227	1.978
10	220	9.285×10^{11}	206	2.451
7	210	8.863	196	2.687
5	201	8.496	188	2.908
2	180	7.610	169	3.507
1	166	6.963	154	4.008

*S.E.M.=standard error of the mean.

Cell survival probabilities for the case of monoenergetic gamma rays of various energies, isotropically incident on the phantom, are shown in Figure 8. The values depicted are in two groups, one for the high energies (3-14 MeV) and one for the low energies (0.1-1.5 MeV). Within each group, the order is not consistent due to complexities in the transport process and, possibly, due to statistical variations from group to group in the Monte Carlo results.

Uncertainties in the extrapolation dose D_o, nominally taken to be 91 centigrays, have been investigated and the results depicted in Figure 9 for incident 1 to 1.5 MeV gamma rays. A change in D_o of 10% in either direction has a substantial effect on cell mortality.

Cell survival probabilities for the case of monoenergetic neutrons of various energies, isotropically incident on the phantom are shown in Figure 10. These results include the contribution on neutron-induced gamma rays produced within the phantom. In this case, the results are well behaved, showing increasing survival with decreasing incident energy. Changes in cell survival in the neutron field caused by variations in D_o and m values are insignificant.

The neutron survival function for marrow is the weakest in terms of the quality of its parameters, since these were derived based on 14 MeV neutron irradiation of mouse marrow and not on heavy ion bombardment as Katz prefers. Thus, the value of D_o is uncertain. Further, according to his publications, Katz assumed an average value of charge which varied uniformly over the track length of the charged particle. This is not correct. A charged particle has an integer number of electrons associated with it at any time. Thus, a computed Z of 0.5 for a proton means that it has an electron associated with it one-half of the time. SAI has taken the position that no ionization can occur while the proton is traveling in the neutral state and that particles having other charge

38

values are affected accordingly. Using the descrete charge or "quantum" model, the survival is much greater than with the old model. This is mainly because of the transport of neutral proton-electron systems over portions of the track length previously assigned a non-zero Z value. All other values of marrow survival from incident neutrons shown in this report have been computed using the quantum model.

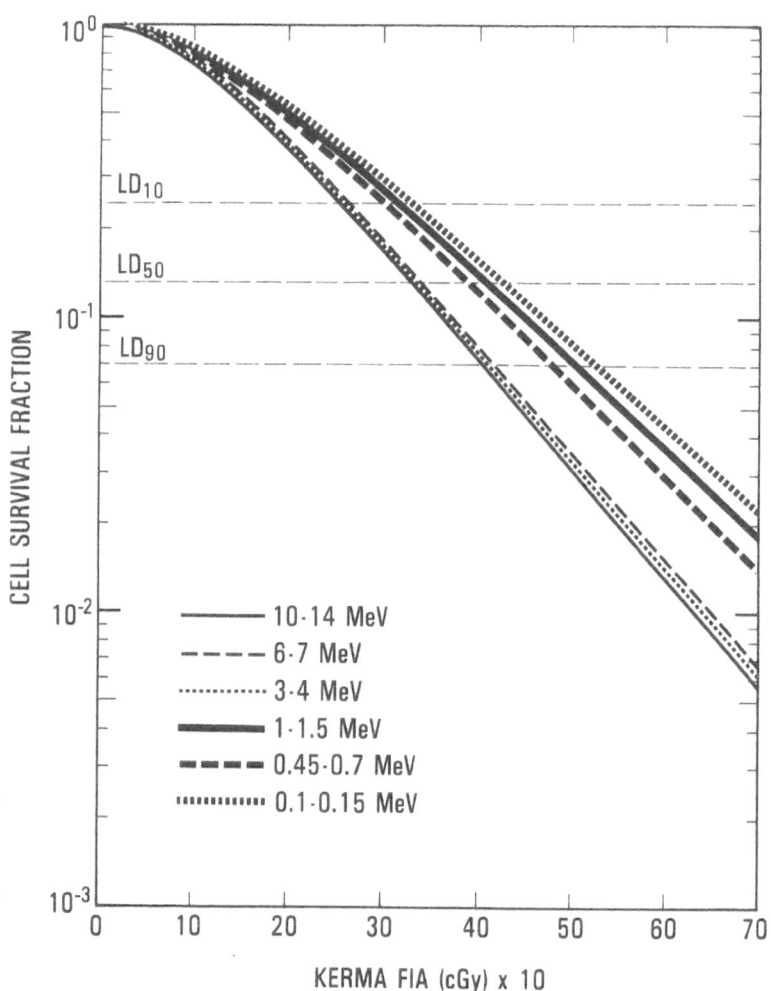

Figure 8.   Bone marrow cell survival following whole-body gamma ray exposure. Light curve: 10-14 MeV (solid), 6-7 MeV (dash), 3-4 MeV (dotted). Heavy curve: 1-1.5 MeV (solid), 0.45-0.7. MeV (dash), 0.1-0.15 MeV (dotted) lines.

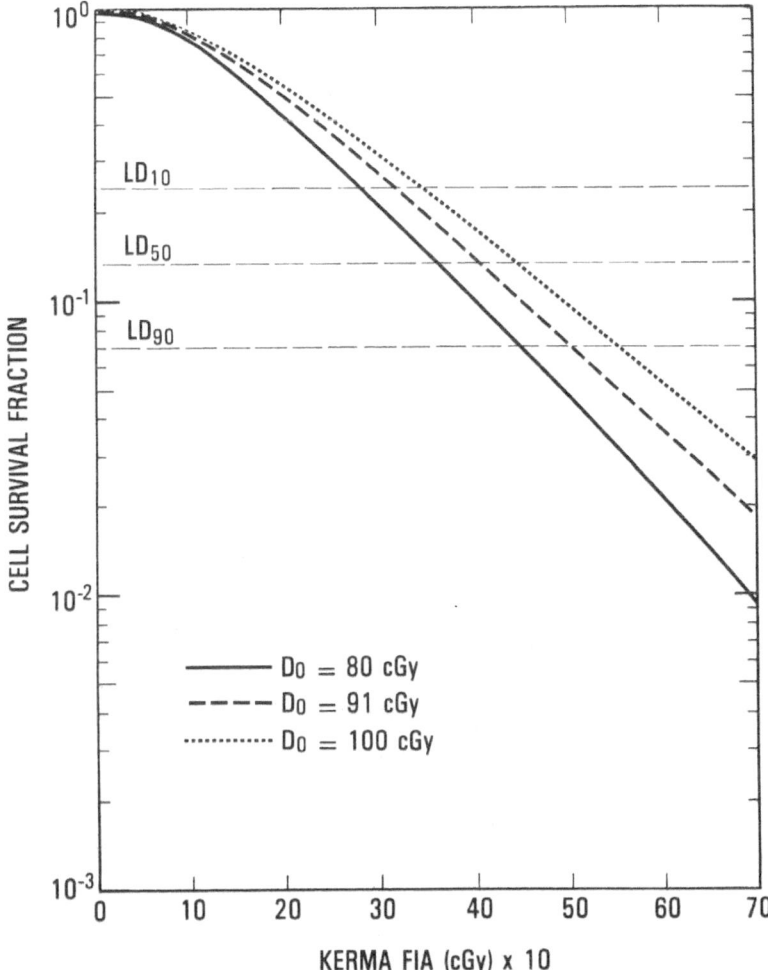

Figure 9. Variation of bone marrow cell survival with D$_o$ for incident 1 to 1.5 MeV gamma rays; Do=80 centigrays (solid), 91 centigrays (dashed), and 100 centigrays (dotted).

The results of computations of cell survival in a tactical weapon radiation field are shown in Figure 11. LD$_{50}$ occurs at free field kerma levels of between 260 and 310 centigrays. Note that the difference between 13% cell survival (LD$_{50}$) and 20% cell survival (LD$_{20}$) is either a matter of the distance required for a 20% change in dose <u>or</u> the direction the person is facing at the time of exposure. This effect is enhanced when the cell survival computation is performed separately for each marrow region instead of for the total marrow as depicted here (2,3).

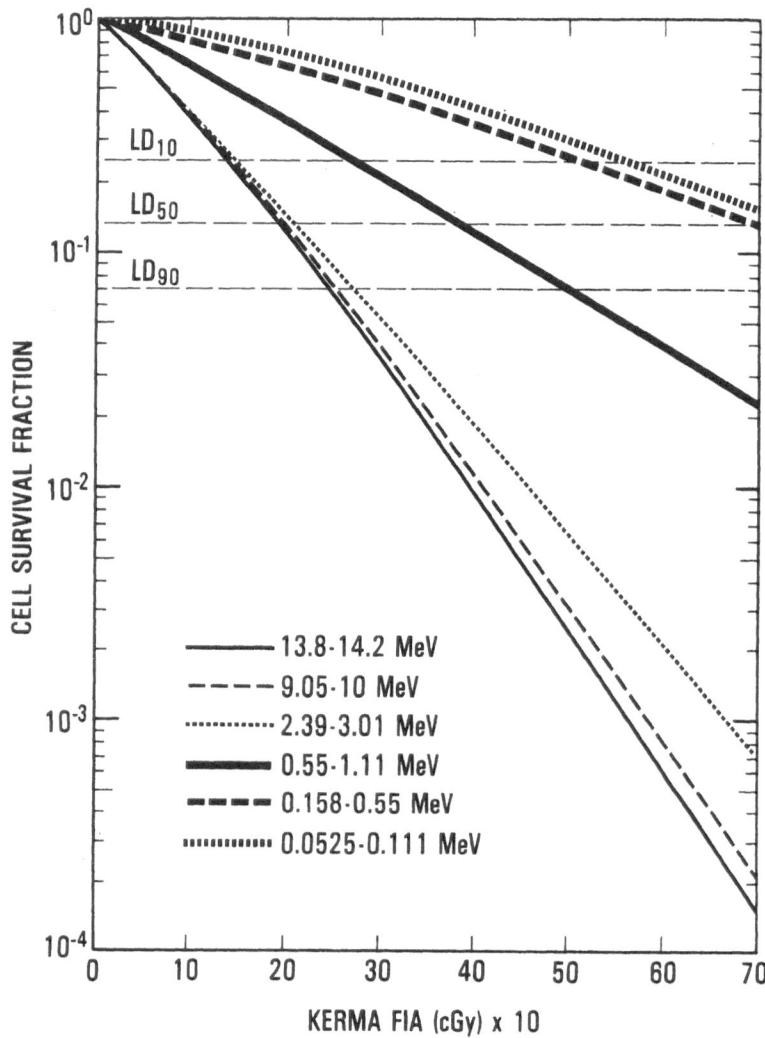

Figure 10. Cell survival from incident neutrons including neutron-induced gamma rays. Light curve: 13.8–14.2 MeV (solid), 9.05–10.0 MeV (dashed), 2.39–3.01 (dotted). Heavy curve: 0.55–1.11 (solid), 0.158–0.55 (dashed), 0.0525–0.111 (dotted).

This communication has illustrated the power of calculational methods in determining fluence, kerma and other quantities at sensitive sites within the human body for a variety of exposure conditions. The computation techniques will shortly be tested experimentally with lab oratory pigs and monkeys. The cell survival/human mortality correlation is expected to be useful in showing the effects of irregular geometry, mixed LET and energy-varying exposure conditions. However, it is important that experiments be performed, using heavy charged particles, to obtain data on which to base σ_o, the sensitive site cross-section, in the Katz model. It is further suggested that future studies of human mortality from radiation exposure be based on the cell survival values which most closely relate to exposure conditions, and not on average kerma values within or without the body.

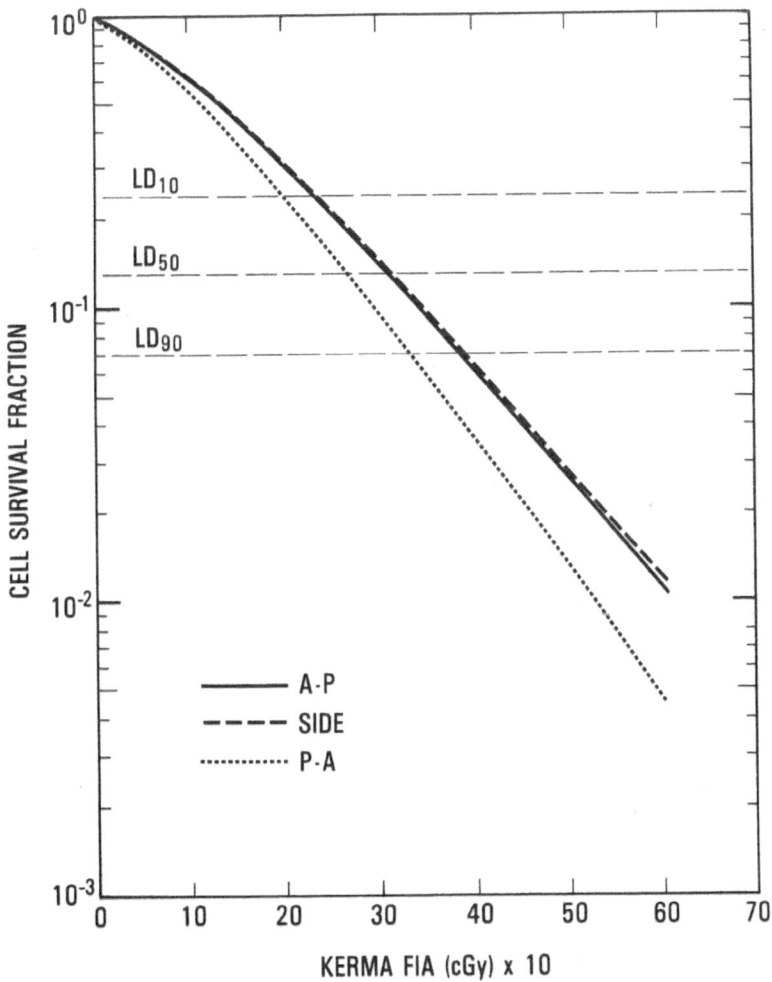

Figure 11. Bone marrow cell survival in the tactical radiation field for different orientations; A-P (solid), side (dashed), P-A (dotted) lines.

References

1. Kaul, D., and Jarka, R. Radiation Dose Deposition in the Active Marrow of Reference Man. DNA 442F, October 1977.

2. Scott, W.H., Jr. and Kaul, D.C., et al., Dosimeter and Bone Marrow Doses in Tactical Nuclear Environments. SAI-133-269-LJ, 15 Feb 1980.

3. Scott, W.H., Jr. and Kaul, D.C. Evaluation of Bone Marrow Cell Survival and Dosimeter Doses in Tactical Nuclear Environments. SAI-133-81-212-LJ, June 1981.

4. Bond, V.P. and Thiessen, J.W., ed., Reevaluations of Dosimetric Factors: Hiroshima and Nagasaki. CONF-810928, U.S. Department of Energy, Oct 1982.

5. Cristy, M. Mathematical Phantoms Representing Children of Various Ages for Use in Estimates of Internal Dose. ORNL/NUREG/TM-367, Oak Ridge National Laboratory, June 1980.

6. Rhoades, W.A., et al. Vehicle Code System (VCS) User's Manual. ORNL-TM-4648, Oak Ridge National Laboratory, August 1974.

7. Katz, R., et al. Inactivation of cells by heavy ion bombardment. Radiation Research 47:402-425 (1971).

8. Katz, R. and Sharma, S. Response of cells to fast neutrons, stopped pions, and heavy ion beams. Nuclear Instruments and Methods III (1973), pp 93-116.

9. Katz, R. and Sharma, S. RBE-dose relations for neutrons and pions. Phys. Med. Biol. 20(3):410-419 (1975).

10. Egbert, S. and Kaul, D.C. MACKSPAR-A Code for Calculating Partial Kerma, Quality and Cell Inactivation Factors. SAI-155-03-0900-01 (1983, to be published).

11. Langham, W.H., ed. Radiobiological Factors in Manned Space Flight. National Academy of Sciences, Publication 1487 (1967).

12. Bond, V.P. and Robinson, C.V. A mortality determination in non-uniform exposures of the mammal. Radiation Research Suppl 7:265-275 (1967).

SUSCEPTIBILITY TO TOTAL BODY IRRADIATION

Vriesendorp, H.M.* and van Bekkum, D.W.**

*Northwestern University, Chicago, IL, USA.
**Radiobiological Institute TNO, Rijswijk, The Netherlands.

Introduction

The susceptibility of human beings to total body irradiation (TBI) can be estimated approximately from experience obtained in nuclear warfare, in accidents with the peaceful use of nuclear energy and in clinical studies employing TBI in cancer patients. This information is documented and reexamined by other authors in these proceedings.
A more precise knowledge of the susceptibility of men to TBI is required for better risk estimates after radiation accidents and for optimizing the therapeutic use of TBI. In this contribution experimental animal data are presented to illustrate models that might be of use in extrapolating finer details of susceptibility of TBI from experimental animals to human individuals. The same issue was addressed in an earlier publication (1). Additional circumstantial evidence in support of the presented models is discussed.

Methods

Animals: CBA T6 mice, Brown Norway x Lewis rats, rhesus monkeys and beagle dogs were used. Male animals were used exclusively in the rat and mouse experiments. Male as well as female dogs and monkeys were included in the tests.

Animal care: Acidified (pH3) drinking water was used for all animals. Reverse barrier nursing, blood component therapy and antibiotics were used for monkeys and dogs only. Subcutaneous Ringer's lactate (75ml/kg/day) was given to dogs and monkeys showing signs of dehydration in the first week after TBI. Microbiologically all animals were "conventional". They were screened for intestinal parasites and Pseudomonas aeroginosa prior to TBI and only used in an experiment if these micro-organisms were absent. Survival was the end point of study for all species. Autopsies were done within 12 hours after death for all dogs and monkeys. Animals were scored as having died from the bone marrow (BM) syndrome on the basis of 1. the observed decrease in their peripheral blood counts after TBI (performed at least 3x a week for all species, except mice), 2. time of death (day 10-30 after TBI) and 3. autopsy results. Animals were scored as having died from the gastrointestinal (GI) syndrome on the basis of 1. death within the first week after TBI, 2. clinical symptomatology-voluminous watery diarrhea 3. autopsy results.

Radiation: Three hundred KV X-rays (10mA, 3.0 mm Cu HVL) were used for TBI in mice, dogs and rhesus monkeys. Dose rates/min. were 1.25 Gy for mice, 0.16 Gy for dogs and 0.06 Gy for monkeys. Dosimetry experiments to verify uniformity of dose have been performed and published previously (2, 3, 4). Rats were irradiated in a ^{157}Cs source with a dose rate of 1.42 Gy/min. A RBE of 0.85 was used to normalize the rat results to the results obtained with orthovoltage X-ray in the other species (2).
Groups of 10 or more (mice, rats) or of 4 or more (dogs, monkeys) were tested for each TBI dose. TBI doses differed by 1.0 Gy.

Bone marrow transplantation: Bone marrow cells were injected i.v. within 30 hours after TBI as a monocellular suspension. The minimal number of bone marrow cells required for rescue of 50% of the animals after TBI was determined by titration of the dose of bone marrow cells. Bone marrow cell doses differed by a factor 2. Animal group size was ten or more in mice and rats and four or more in dogs and monkeys.

Results

The LD_{50} for the bone marrow (BM) syndrome and the gastrointestinal (GI) syndrome was determined in all four species. In addition supralethal TBI in the range between 7.5 Gy (dogs) and 9.0 Gy (mice) was used to establish the number of autologous or isogeneic bone marrow cells required for "rescue" or lasting hemopoietic reconstitution in 50% of the animals. Results are summarized in table 1.

Table 1

Toxicity of TBI and Bone Marrow Cell Dose Required for Rescue

Species (body weight) in kg; BSA in m^2	LD_{50} GI Syndrome in Gy	LD_{50} BM Syndrome in Gy	Autologous or Isogeneic Rescue Dose (cells x 10^6) Per Kg Body Weight	Per m^2 BSA
Mouse (.025;.0075)	12.5	7.00	2.0	6.5
Rat (.2;.030)	11.5	6.75	3.8	24.2
Rhesus Monkey (2.6;.230)	9.5	5.25	7.5	80.0
Dog (12.0;.550)	8.5	3.70	17.5	445.0

^{2}The bone marrow rescue dose is expressed per kg body weight or per m^2 body surface area (BSA). Values of BSA for the different species were obtained from the formulae published by Freireich et al. (5). The larger species are more susceptible to GI and BM toxicity than the smaller species. Individualized blood product support antibiotics and fluid replacement were only given to dogs and monkeys. Without this extra care the LD_{50} for BM and GI syndrome would be approximately 1.5 Gy lower (Unpublished observations). A negative correlation is present between the LD_{50} for the BM syndrome and the bone marrow rescue dose. Thus if a species has a low LD_{50} for the BM syndrome, many bone marrow cells are needed for rescue after supralethal TBI. The correlation coefficient is higher if the bone marrow rescue dose is expressed per kilogram body weight than if the rescue is expressed per body surface area (.99 and .89 respectively). Both correlation coefficients are statistically significant at a p value of $<$.05 (figure 4).

Possible explanations of results

Studies of Bond and coworkers (6, 7) have shown that with the exception of ultra high dose TBI ($>$ 10.000 Gy) the toxicity of TBI is due to disturbances in two self renewal systems, the hemopoietic system and the gastrointestinal mucosa. Self renewal systems contain three compartments, i.e. stem cells, differentiating cells and functional end cells. The stem cells are the most radiosensitive and dose limiting cells. The end cells are hardly influenced by the radiation. Radiation induced deficits in the stem cell compartment will cause symptoms by not replacing end cells. Lack of platelets and white cells mucosa will cause losses in body fluids and electrolytes. The following simplification will be introduced. In properly controlled animal studies extraneous influences are excluded and survival after TBI is dependent only on the number of surviving stem cells and differences in susceptibility to TBI between different experimental animal species will have to be explained in differences between stem cells.

GI Syndrome: Previously, other authors have shown that the interval between TBI and death for the GI syndrome after TBI, is independent of surviving crypt stem cells and dependent on the transit time of the crypt cells to the intestinal villus tip (9). In conventional animals the GI syndrome occurs in the first week after TBI. It seems reasonable to assume that the length of the GI tract (small intestines) is positively correlated with the number of crypt stem cells. If length of the GI tract is expressed by kilogram body weight or BSA the GI tract is longer in herbivores (mice, rats) than in omnivores (monkeys) and is shortest in carnivores (dogs). Thus dogs would be most susceptible to the GI syndrome, because they have less crypt stem cells than the other species. A certain minimum surface of GI mucosa is needed to reabsorb the intraluminal fluids and electrolytes. The critical low number of surviving crypt stem cells would be reached after lower doses of TBI in dogs than in other species. This explanation is compatible with the early observation that shielding of small sections of the distal small intestine can increase the LD_{50} for the GI syndrome (8). Extrapolation of the hypothesis to men (omnivores) would predict the LD_{50} for the GI syndrome after single fraction TBI to be similar to the one found in rhesus monkeys, i.e. equivalent to $\pm$ 9.5 Gy 300 kV x-ray (10).

BM syndrome: Hemopoietic cells that are not stem cells cannot make self copies. They can only differentiate into end cells of one of the hemopoietic sublines (erythrocyte, granulocyte, platelet or lymphocyte). Transfusions of end cells loose effectiveness quickly when used repeatedly and can prevent symptoms of bone marrow cells deficits for short periods of time only. Thus, hemopoietic stem cells (HSC) are crucial to survival after a LD_{50} TBI dose or after a supralethal TBI dose and a bone marrow transplant because they are the only cells that can provide a lasting regeneration of all hemopoietic sublines.

Three different theoretical models can be proposed to explain the results summarized in table 1.

1. Kinetic differences in the hemopoietic system of the investigated species. The marrow transit time (time that the HSC needs to develop in critical end cell) and the survival time in the peripheral blood of those end cells, that are critical for survival, are the variables that influence the LD_{50} for the BM syndrome and the number of bone marrow cells required for rescue.

2. All four species have the same number of HSC per kilogram body weight. Their HSC differ in radiosensitivity.

3. The reverse of 2. HSC in all four species have the same radiosensitivity. Species differ in the number of HSC per kilogram body weight.

The requirements to fulfil possibility 1 are illustrated by examples of theoretical extreme situations in figures 1 and 2. The initial horizontal lines of end cell levels in the peripheral blood shown in the figures reflect the marrow transit time, i.e. the time it takes a HSC to develop into an end cell. The subsequent downward slopes reflect the survival time of end cells in the peripheral blood. The reoccurence of end cells is dependent on the marrow transit time and number of HSC that survived (after LD_{50} TBI) or that was transplanted (after supralethal TBI). In the figures the sum of disappeared and regenerated end cells is shown. The wavy line in the figures indicates a critical end level. Below this level chances for survival decrease. The longer an end cell curve is below this "survival" level, the higher the chance for death from the BM syndrome. Figure 1A illustrates that the length of the marrow transit time does not influence the LD_{50} for TBI. The end cell levels change in a similar pattern for long and short transit times. In contrast, species with end cells, that survive long, will have a higher LD_{50} for TBI than species with end cells that show a short survival (figure 2A). After a supralethal TBI dose ($> LD_{100}$) the disappearance of end cells is less dependent on the marrow transit time of stem cells as more cells in the differentiation compartment are inactivated by TBI. Therefore, a short interval between stem cell and end cell will be advantageous after supralethal TBI and bone marrow transplantation as it decreases the length of time that end cells are dangerously low (figure 1B). For the same reason a longer survival time of critical end cells would improve survival after supralethal TBI and bone marrow transplantation (figure 2B). In summary the negative correlation between bone marrow rescue dose and LD_{50} for the BM syndrome can only be explained if species with a high LD_{50} have critical end cells (platelets, granulocytes) that survive long and a marrow transit time that is short. Vice versa species with a low LD_{50} would have a long marrow transit time and critical end cells that survive for only a brief period. The available evidence indicates that only small differences exist

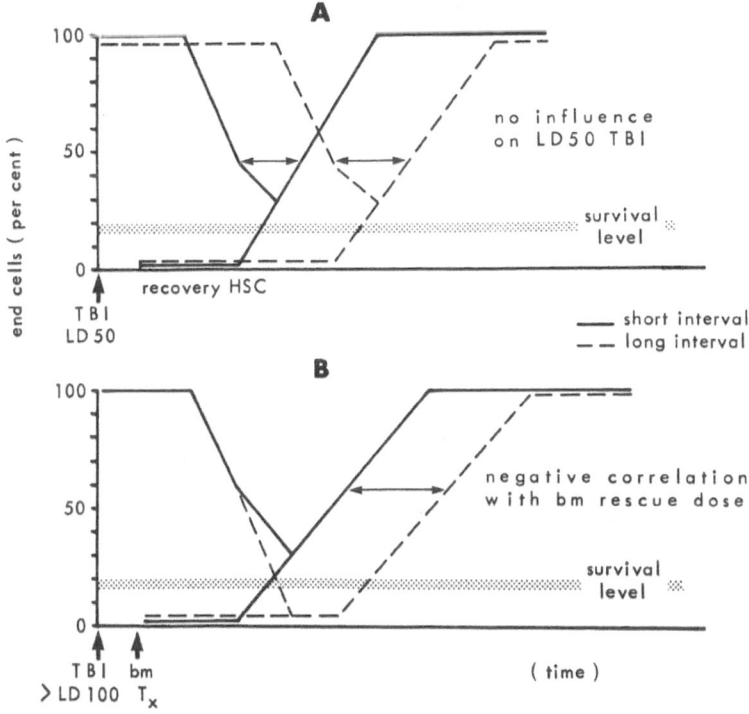

Figure 1.
Influence of Variations in Marrow Transit Time (Interval Stem Cell-End Cell) on LD_{50} TBI (A) and Bone Marrow Rescue Dose (B) Between Species.

48

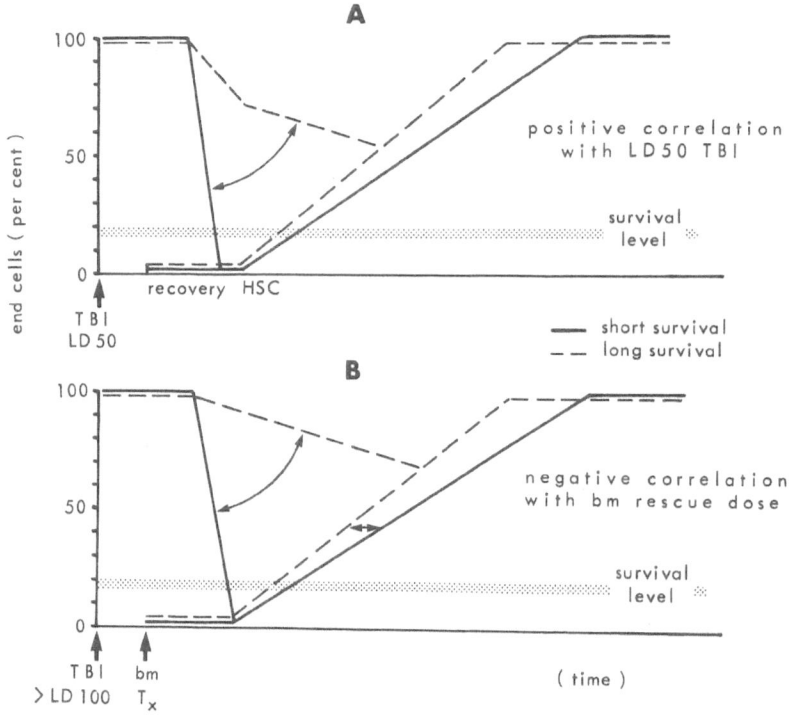

Figure 2.
Influence of Variations in Survival (Life Span) of End Cells on LD$_{50}$ TBI (A) and Bone Marrow Rescue Dose (B) Between Species.

between species in these parameters (11). The disappearance of granulocytes and platelets after a dose of supralethal TBI is a reflection of the same two parameters, i.e. survival of end cells and to a lesser degree marrow transit time. Granulocytes and platelets disappear at the same rate after TBI in all four species.
The observations for rats and dogs in this study are given in figure 3. The above indicates that differences in kinetics of the hemopoietic system cannot explain the differences in susceptibility to TBI.

For possibility 2 the assumption is made that all species have the same number of HSC per kilogram body weight. The fractional survival of HSC at the LD$_{50}$ TBI dose should be the same in all species. In mice, radiation survival of HSC has been determined using the spleen colony assay (12) and a low extrapolation number and D$_0$ were found. In this paper the following

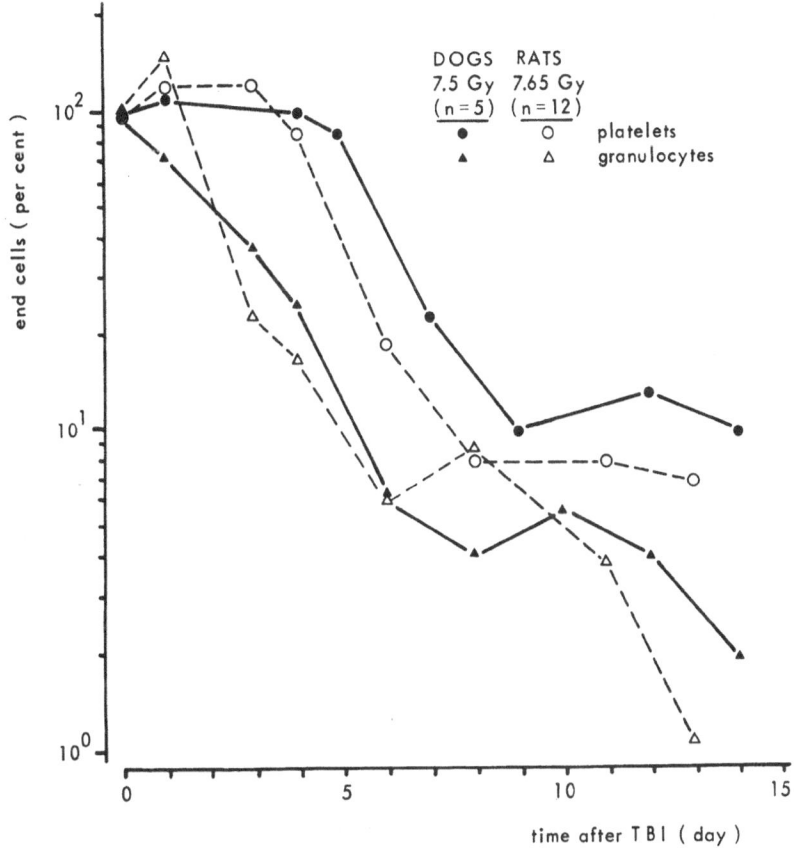

Figure 3.
Disappearance of Blood Cells After Supralethal Total Body Irradiation.

radiation survival parameters are used for HSC: n = 1 and $D_0 = .60$ Gy. This gives a fractional HSC survival of approximately 1×10^{-5} at the LD_{50} of mice in table 1 (7.0 Gy). In dogs and monkeys to obtain the same fractional survival after 3.70 Gy and 5.25 Gy respectively, one would have to postulate unrealistically small D_0, i.e. .35 Gy for dogs and .49 Gy for monkeys. Another consequence of the assumption that species have the same number of HSC per kilogram body weight is that they would require the same number of bone marrow cells per kilogram for rescue after supralethal TBI. The latter is obviously not the case (table 1). The above eliminates possibility 2 as explanation of the observations made.

The last possible explanation (3) i.e., differences in HSC concentrations between species, assumes the same radiosensitivity of HSC in each species. To test this hypothesis the number of HSC that survives a LD_{50} TBI has to be computed. Additional data needed to perform such computations are: 1. total numbers of bone marrow cells per species, 2. the fraction of i.v. injected HSC that "homes" into the bone marrow and spleen to start hemopoietic regeneration and 3. the D_0 and n of the radiation survival curve of HSC. Pegg has reviewed the total number of bone marrow cells per species (13). Van Bekkum and coworkers have estimated the homing fraction of i.v. injected mouse HSC on the basis of retransplantation experiments to be $\pm$ 0.3 (14). Under the conditions postulated the total number of bone marrow cells needed for rescue (table 2) divided by the total number of bone marrow cells provides an estimate of fractional HSC survival after a LD_{50} TBI dose. A significant linear correlation (r = 0.99) is found between LD_{50} TBI dose and fractional HSC survival of the four species investigated (1). This indicates that the assumption of similar radiation sensitivity of HSC of the different species is not unreasonable. Computations were made using a n = 1 and a D_0 = .60 Gy for HSC in all species as these parameters gave the highest correlation coefficient. Those values are similar to estimates obtained by other workers by other methods in mice (2, 12). In table 2 the number of HSC surviving a LD_{50} TBI are compared to the number of HSC required for 50% rescue after supralethal TBI. Hypothesis 3 requires that these numbers are approximately equal. For mice, rats and monkeys, this is indeed the case. In dogs a four fold difference is found.

Table 2

Comparison of Number of Bone Marrow Cells Surviving LD_{50} Dose of TBI with Number of Bone Marrow Cells Required to Rescue 50% of the Animals after Supralethal TBI

Species	Total Number of Bone Marrow Cells x 10^9*	Number of Bone Marrow Cells Surviving LD_{50} TBI x 10^8**	Number of Bone Marrow Cells Needed for Rescue x 10^6***
Mouse	1	0.010	0.015
Rat	5.9	0.083	0.167
Rhesus Monkey	62.4	10.4	6.0
Dog	120	264.0	70.0

  * Pegg 1966, with exception of the dog (13).
 ** Assumption of radiation survival curve with n = 1 and D_0 = .60 Gy.
*** Total number of injected cells x homing fraction (= 0.3) + autologous cells surviving 8.0 Gy TBI.

The precision of the comparison is influenced by several factors. The homing fraction of intravenously infused bone marrow cells is known only for mice. The LD_{50} for dogs and rhesus monkeys are less accurate because of greater dosimetric problems and less animals per points. If the LD_{50} for dogs is 10% higher than the one observed and this is within the margins of dosimetric error in the large, inhomogenous volume of the dog the differences between the last two columns in table 2 would be only a factor 2 for dogs. Alternatively a slightly lower D_0 for canine HSC (approx. .55

instead of .60 Gy) or a higher homing fraction would clean up the difference.

The preceding paragraphs indicate that the differences in suscepti-bility between species for hematological toxicity of TBI are best explained by assuming high concentrations of HSC in radioresistant species and low concentrations of HSC in radiosensitive species. This is the only model that explains effectively that radioresistant species need more bone marrow cells for rescue. In addition the HSC of the dog might be slightly more radiosensitive, but the margins of error in dosimetry and LD_{50} determi-nations in this species are currently too large for a final decision on that issue.

Additional arguments for species differences in HSC concentrations

Freireich et al. (5) have compared the effects of eighteen different chemotherapeutic agents in the same species as the ones analyzed in this TBI study. They found that toxicity occurs at the same dose level in species, if the dose is expressed per m^2 BSA. Correction factors were needed if doses were expressed per kg body weight. Then small sized species tolerated higher drug doses than larger species. A theoretical example is given in table 3.

Table 3

Comparison of Toxicity of Chemotherapeutic Agents in Different Species

Species	Equivalent* Toxic Dose per m^2 BSA	Equivalent* Toxic Dose per Kg Body Weight	Relative** HSC Concentration per Kg; per BSA	
Mouse	1	12	10	120
Rat	1	7	6.7	32
Rhesus Monkey	1	3	2.7	9.7
Dog	1	2	1.1	1.7
Man	1	1	1	1

* Freireich et al. 1966, Cancer Chemotherapy Reports 50, 219.
** The number of bone marrow cells per kilogram body weight or BSA estimated to rescue 50% of lethally irradiated humans being divided by the number of bone marrow cells required to rescue 50% of lethally irradiated individuals of a given species.

Toxicity results are expressed in drug dose per m^2 BSA, or per kilo-gram body weight. A third and fourth column of results provide a measure of the relative hemopoietic stem cell concentration in the various species. These values were obtained for each species by dividing the estimate of the human bone marrow rescue cell dose per kilogram or BSA (see next paragraph) by the bone marrow rescue cell dose per kilogram or BSA of each species. It is clear that toxicity differences are well explained by differences in HSC concentration between species if bone marrow rescue dose is expressed in kilogram body weight (column 2 and 3). Bone marrow rescue dose expressed per BSA does not correlate with equivalent toxic dose of chemotherapeutic agents expressed per BSA (columns 1 and 4 in table 3). The tolerance of small animals for chemotherapy appears to be greater because they have more hemopoietic stem cells per kilogram body weight.

In the past the results in the first column of table 3 have led to the recommendation to express the dose of chemotherapeutic agents by m^2 BSA as the same dose could be used for all species (5). Studies of domesticated animals had shown that the basic metabolic rate was the same in all species if expressed per m^2 BSA and different if expressed per kg body weight (15, 16). Drug elimination correlates better with BSA than kg body weight. Peak drug serum levels correlate better with kg body weight than BSA (17). For most of the current chemotherapeutic agents (17 out of the 18 drugs reviewed by Freirech et al.) hematological toxicity is dose limiting. BSA or basic metabolic rate does not have a straight forward correlation to the dose limiting target cell, the HSC. The uniform equivalent toxic dose of chemotherapeutic agents for all species when expressed per m^2 is only an artifact because the ratio body weight/BSA is smaller in smaller animals. This will give lower drug doses in smaller animals if doses are expressed per BSA and obscure the real differences that are found if results are expressed per kg body weight. An additional advantage of body weight over BSA is that the former is easier to measure. The practical significance of changing the denominator in expressing the drug dose from m^2 BSA to kg body weight is limited for adult human cancer patients. After extensive phase I studies an optimal total drug dose will be known. It is inconsequential whether this drug dose is divided by m^2 BSA or kg body weight. Another argument in favor of BSA as unit for drug dose, has been that an identical dose can be used in young and old individuals of the same species (15). The same argumentation as followed for the interspecies drug comparison can be used to challenge this concept. However, for this situation the data in experimental animals are very limited. Younger, lighter individuals might be able to tolerate more drug because they have more HSC per kilogram body weight than older, heavier individuals of the same species. This should be reflected in the susceptibility to TBI. In dogs, sheep and mice the LD_{50} for TBI is higher in young than in old animals (18, 19). However, the reverse has been found in rats and Chinese hamsters (20, 21). To our knowledge a quantitative comparison of rescue potential of bone marrow cells of young and old bone marrow donors has not been made so far. Younger animals could also end up having more HSC than older animals if their HSC concentration is the same but the bone marrow cellularity per kilogram body weight is higher. Obviously, the experimental animal data are incomplete and insufficient to decide the issue either way. In human pediatric patients problems might occur if adult drug doses are used for extrapolation to drug doses in children. A hypothetical example is given in table 4. Children will receive higher total drug doses if m^2 BSA instead of kg body weight is used for dose determination. Increased myelosuppression has been described in neonates and very young infants with Wilms's tumor receiving actinomycin D, adriamycin and vincristine per m^2 BSA. The National Wilms' Tumor Study Committee has recommended to reduce the dosage levels in infants 11 months of age (approx. 8 kg) or younger by

50% (22). This dose reduction is very similar to the one shown in table 4 (column 5) if kg body weight is used for determination of drug dose. The general impression has been that older children can tolerate higher doses of chemotherapy than adults (23). Notable exceptions are caused by agents, that do not have hemopoietic stem cells as the dose limiting target cells. Children are more susceptible to anthracycline induced cardiomyopathy (24) and methotrexate neurotoxicity than adults (25). This indicates that the most useful expression of drug dose is in terms of dose limiting target cells. The collective evidence appears to indicate that kg body weight is well correlated with the amount of HSC and a better unit for dosing of hematotoxic drugs than BSA.

TABLE 4

Differences in Dose of Chemotherapeutic Agents if Expressed per Kg Body Weight or Body Surface Area for Young Patients.

Kg Body Weight	m^2 BSA	Total Dose BSA Prescription	Total dose per Kg Body Weight Prescription	Difference between BSA & Kg Body Weight Prescription
70 (Adult)	1.85	1.85	1.85	0
40	1.35	1.35	1.06	−21%
20	.80	.80	.53	−34%
8	.40	.40	.21	−48%
3	.20	.20	.08	−60%

Assumption: optimal dose of hypothetical drug is 1 g/m^2 in an adult. This will give a drug dose of 0.0264 g/kg. Lower total doses of drug will be given in younger patients if kg body weight is taken as the basis for drug prescription.

Extrapolations to humans of susceptibility to TBI and autologous or isogeneic bone marrow transplantation

The model outlined offers predictions for bone marrow rescue dose and LD_{50} for man. The assumptions are that body weight is correlated with HSC concentration and that HSC concentrations determine LD_{50} and bone marrow rescue dose of TBI. Figure 4 shows the extrapolated correlation between body weight and bone marrow rescue dose and between BSA and bone marrow rescue dose. Kilogram body weight shows a higher correlation with bone marrow rescue dose than m^2 BSA (corr. coeff. of .99 versus .89). The significant correlation between BSA and bone marrow rescue cell dose can be explained by its relation to body weight (roughly BSA = k x kg 2/3, in which k is a constant that differs per age group and species (26).

54

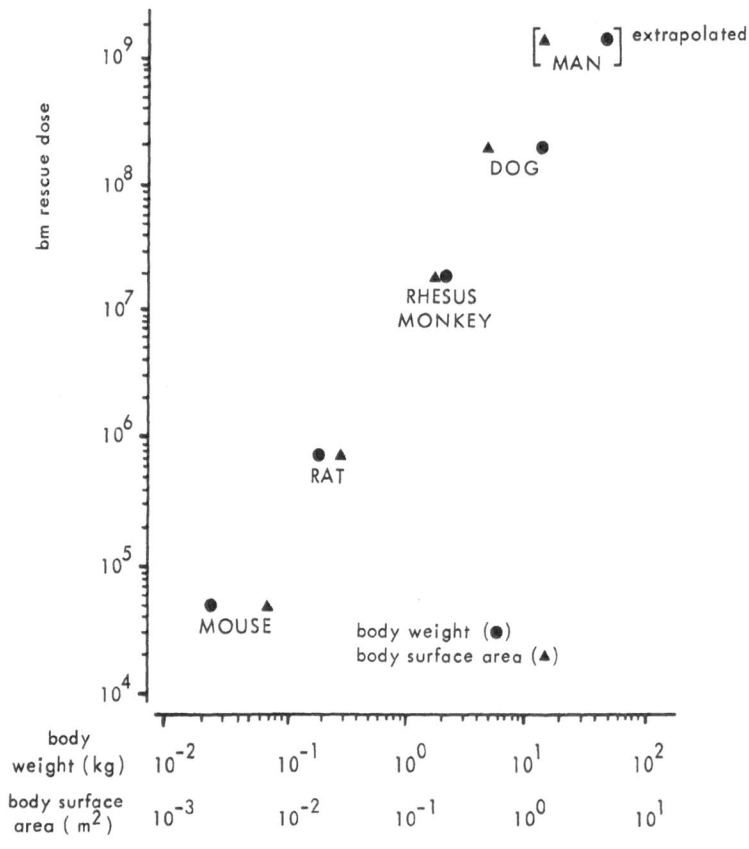

Figure 4.
Correlation Between Body Weight (●) or Body Surface Area (▲) and Minimal
Bone Marrow Rescue Dose After LD_{100} TBI.

For 70 kg men, a bone marrow dose of 2×10^7/kg body weight would be
lifesaving in 50% of the cases. In animals a doubling of the 50% rescue
dose generally gives a 100% rescue dose. Thus 4×10^7 <u>autologous</u> bone
marrow cells per kg body weight would be the minimal rescue cell dose after
lethal TBI in man. In man the minimum rescue cell dose for HLA identical,
<u>allogeneic</u> bone marrow cells is approximately 1×10^8/kg body weight (27).
Above this dose hemopoietic recovery is the rule. Below this dose 2 out of
seven patients did not achieve hemopoietic recovery (10). In comparisons
of autologous and histocompatible allogeneic bone marrow transplants in
mice and dogs (28, 29) approximately four times as many allogeneic bone
marrow cells were required for rescue in both species. If the same holds
for man the above indicates that the human allogeneic bone marrow transplant data are in agreement with the estimate obtained from extrapolations

from the experimental animal data.
The LD_{50} for the bone marrow syndrome after TBI in man can be extrapolated from the proposed model if the following assumptions are made.
1. The human HSC has a D_0 of .60 Gy and a n of 1.
2. The total number of human bone marrow cells is approximately 10^{10}/kg
   body weight (13).
3. The homing fraction of human bone marrow cells is approximately 0.3.
The fraction of bone marrow cells required for 50% rescue is the same as
the fraction of bone marrow cells surviving a LD_{50} TBI (table 2). The
former can be computed with the data provided for man as approximately 6 x
10^{-4} (0.3 x 2 x 10^7/10^{10}). On a dose fractional survival curve this
surviving fraction would occur after a TBI dose of approximately 4.5 Gy
calculated as follows:

$$\text{surviving fraction} = 6 \times 10^{-4} = e^{-\frac{LD50}{Do}}$$

$$\text{Ln } 6 \times 10^{-4} = -\frac{LD50}{0.6} = -7.42$$

$$LD_{50} = 7.42 \times 0.6 \text{ Gy} = 4.5 \text{ Gy}.$$

This is similar to estimates for the LD_{50} of man derived from nuclear
warfare, radiation accidents and therapeutic TBI in man (see articles by
Smith and Baverstock in this volume).

Perspectives

Therapeutic TBI, such as used for allogeneic or autologous bone marrow
transplantation in man, is a very toxic procedure. The influence of
radiation modality, dose rate, fractionation, inhomogeneous dose, shielding
of critical organs remains to be defined for the relevant endpoints in man
i.e. acute effects, late effects, immunosuppression and tumor eradication.
Experimental resolution of these open questions is difficult to obtain in
man for obvious reasons (ethical constraints, the number of variables
involved).
In this contribution we suggest that the acute affects of TBI in man
can be extrapolated from results in experimental animals, if differences in
dose limiting self renewal systems between species are taken into account.
Experimental animal models are less predictable for late effects, immunosuppressive effects or tumor eradication in human patients. This
unsatisfactory situation might be resolved by the development of new models
for these endpoints, similar in nature to the ones proposed for acute TBI
effects. The reported results as well as an analysis of data from the
literature available appear to support the model proposed. Stem cells
determine the susceptibility to TBI and the concentration and/or total
amount of stem cells differ between species. In the future when stem cells
can be identified quantitatively in vitro in all species and this appears
to be close to reality for HSC, the proposed model could be tested and
applied more rigorously. This development would also resolve the problem of
the determination of stem cell reserve in diseased or previously treated
individuals. In healthy individuals length of the small intestines and
kilogram body weight appears to be the best currently available correlates
for the number of crypt stem cells and hemopoietic stem cells respectively.
These stem cells are also of major importance in the prediction of GI or
bone marrow toxicity to cancer chemotherapeutic agents.

References

1. H.M. Vriesendorp and D.W. van Bekkum. Role of total body irradiation in conditioning for bone marrow transplantation. In: Immunobiology of bone marrow transplantation. (Eds. S. Thierfelder, H. Rodt and H.J. Kolb). Supplement to Blut, Springer Verlag, Berlin, Heidelberg, 1980, p. 349.

2. J.J. Broerse, A.C. Engels, P. Lelieveld, L.M. van Putten, W. Duncan, D. Greene, J.B. Massay, C.W. Gilbert, J.H. Hendry and A. Howard. The survival of colony forming units in mouse bone marrow after in vivo irradiation with D-T neutrons, x- and gammaradiation. Int. J. Radiat. Biol., 19, (1971) p. 101.

3. J.J. Broerse, D.W. van Bekkum, C.F. Hollander and J.A.G. Davids. Mortality of monkeys after exposure to fission neutrons and the effect of autologous bone marrow transplantation. Int. J. Radiat. Biol., 34, (1978) p. 253.

4. H.M. Vriesendorp and C. Zurcher. Late effects of total body irradiation in dogs treated with bone marrow transplantation, p. 71. In: Effects after therapeutic whole body irradiation, Report EUR 8078. (Eds. T.M. Fliedner, W. Gossner and G. Patrick), Commission of the European Communities, Luxembourg, 1982.

5. E.J. Freireich, E.A. Gehan, D.P. Rall, L.H. Smith and H.E. Skipper. Quantitative comparison of toxicity of anticancer agents in mouse, rat, dog, monkey and man. Cancer Chemotherapy Report, 50 (1966) p. 219.

6. V.P. Bond, T.M. Fliedner and J.O. Archambeau. Mammalian Radiation Lethality. A disturbance in cellular kinetics, Academic Press, New York, London, 1968.

7. V.P. Bond and T. Sugahara (eds.). Comparative cellular and species radiosensitivity. William and Wilkins Co., Baltimore, 1969.

8. M.N. Swift and S.T. Taketa. Modification of acute intestinal radiation syndrome through shielding. Am. J. Physiol., 185 (1956) p. 85.

9. R.J.M. Fry, A.B. Reiskin, W. Kisieleski, A. Sallese and E. Staffeldt. Radiation effects and cell renewal in rodent intestine. Comparative cellular and species radiosensitivity. (Eds. V.P. Bond and T. Sugahara), Williams & Wilkins Co., Baltimore, 1969.

10. J.J. Broerse and D.W. van Bekkum. Mortality of monkeys after exposure to fission neutrons and the effect of autologous bone marrow transplantation. Int. J. Radiat. Biol., 34 (1978) p. 253-264.

11. T.M. Fliedner. A cytokinetic comparison of hematological consequences of radiation exposure in different mammalian species. Comparative cellular and species radiosensitivity. (Eds. V.P. Bond and T. Sugahara), Williams & Wilkins Co., Baltimore, 1969.

12. J.E. Till and E.A. McCulloch. A direct measurement of the radiation sensitivity of normal mouse bone marrow cells. Radiat. Res., 14 (1961) p. 213.

13. D.E. Pegg. Bone marrow transplantation. Lloyd Luke Ltd. London: 1966.

14. D.W. van Bekkum, B. Löwenberg and H.M. Vriesendorp. Bone marrow transplantation. In: Immunological engineering MTP Press. (Eds D.W. Hirsch), Lancaster, England, 1978, p. 179.

15. D. Pinkel. The use of body surface areas as a criterion of drug dosage in cancer chemotherapy. Cancer Res., 18 (1958) p. 853.

16. M. Kleiber. Body size and metabolic rate physiological reviews. Volume 27 (1947) p. 511.

17. L.B. Mellet. The constancy of the product of concentration and time. Chapter 17. In: Antineoplastic and immunosuppressive agents. Handebuch der experimentellen Pharmakologie. (Eds. A.C. Sartorelli and D.G. Johns), Springer-Verlag, Berlin, volume 38, 1975.

18. R.J. Garner, R.D. Phemister, G.M. Angleton, A.C. Lee and R.W. Thomassen. Effect of age on the acute lethal response of the beagle to cobalt 60 gamma radiation. Radiol. Res., 58 (1974) p. 190.

19. P.B. Roberts and A.T. Pfeffer. Evidence for a decreased susceptibility to acute radiation lethality in young lambs (Personal communication).

20. U. Reincke, J. Mellman and E. Goldmann. Variations in Radioresistance of rats during the period of growth. Int. J. Radiol. Biol., 15 (1967) p. 127.

21. B.C. Ward, J.R. Childress and G.L. Jessup. Effect of age on radiation mortality in the Chinese hamster. Radiol. Res., 20 (1963) p. 288.

22. S.E. Siegel and R.G. Moran. Problems in the chemotherapy of cancer in the neonate. Am. J. Rad. Hem. Onc., 3 (1981) p. 287.

23. W.A. Bleyer. Delayed toxicities of chemotherapy on childhood tissues. Front. Radiat. Ther. Onc., 16 (1982) p. 50.

24. W.A. Bleyer and T.W. Griffin. White matter necrosis, mineralizing microangiopathy and intellectual abilities in survival of childhood leukemia; Association with central nervous system irradiation and methotrexate therapy. In: Radiation damage to the nervous system. (Eds. Gilber and Kagan), Raven Press, New York, 1980.

25. D.D. van Hoff, M. Rozencweig, M. Layard, M. Slavik and F.M. Muggia. Daunomycin induced cardiotoxicity in children and adults. Am. J. Med., p. 62-200 (1977).

26. P. Quiring. Surface area determination. In: Medical Physics, I. (Eds. Glasser), Chicago Year Book Publishers, Inc., 1955.

27. E.D. Thomas, C.A. Buckner, M. Benaji, R.A. Clift, A. Fefer, N. Flournoy, B.W. Goodell, R.O. Hickman, K.G. Lerner, P.E. Neiman, G.E. Sale, G.E. Sanders, J. Singer, M. Stevens, R. Storb and P.L. Weiden. One hundred patients with acute leukemia treated by chemotherapy total body irradiation and allogeneic bone marrow transplantation. Blood, 49 (1977) p. 511.

28. H.M. Vriesendorp, B. Löwenberg, T.P. Visser, S. Knaan and D.W. van Bekkum. Influence of genetic resistance and silica particles on survival after bone marrow transplantation. Transplant. Proc., 8 (1976), p. 483.

29. H.M. Vriesendorp, W.M. Klapwijk, P.J. Heidt, B. Hogeweg and D.W. van Bekkum. Factors controlling the engraftment of transplanted dog bone marrow cells. Tissue Antigens, 20 (1982) p. 63.

ACUTE LETHALITY - THE HEMOPOIETIC SYNDROME IN DIFFERENT SPECIES

A. L. Carsten

Medical Department
Brookhaven National Laboratory
Upton, New York 11973

Introduction

The following presentation will consist of two segments. The first is a general consideration of the hemopoietic syndrome and its variation among animal species. The second portion includes a discussion of studies done within the Medical and Biology Departments at Brookhaven aimed at gaining a better understanding of the hemopoietic syndrome and its modification in mammalian systems.

Species Differences in LD_{50}

The nature and cause for differences in species radiosensitivity continue to be topics of interest for radiobiologists as attested to by the multitude of individual papers, numerous review papers, previous workshops and the convening of this symposium. Principle among earlier discussions of this subject are; the International Seminar on "Comparative Cellular and Species Radiosensitivity in Animals - Cellular Kinetics in Hematopoietic and Gastrointestinal Death," (see Bond and Sugahara 1969), and the text "Mammalian Radiation Lethality" (Bond, Fliedner and Archambeau 1965). Much of the basic information contained in the following paragraphs are taken from these sources as well as from the papers by Ainsworth et al., 1965; Ainsworth and Leong, 1966; Ainsworth and Mitchell, 1967; Hanks, et al., 1966; Holloway, et al., 1968; Leong, et al., 1964; Leong, et al., 1967; Nachwey, et al., 1967; Paige et al., 1968; Nelson, 1969, Alpen, 1967.

For the mammalian species examined to date, the average $LD_{50/30}$ values range from approximately 150 rads to 1500 rads (Table 1). As noted by Bond and Robertson (1957), the mammalian species tend to fall into two broad categories, all large species having a relatively low LD_{50} (150 to 265 rads) with the smaller species ranging from approximately 540 to 1520 rads. However, some exceptions to this include the monkey, the guinea pig and the marmoset. Bond has suggested that these exceptions may be due to either bacterial infections in the guinea pig or parasitic infections in marmosets and monkeys.

Hemopoietic Syndrome

It was early recognized that an inverse relationship existed between the size of whole body x-ray exposure and survival time in the mammalian species. It was similarly apparent that death during the acute phase (for most mammals

Research supported by the U.S. Department of Energy under Contract No. DE-AC02-76CH00016.

Species	Type of radiation	LD$_{50/30}$ days (rads)	Mean survival time (days)
LD$_{50/30}$ for Various Species Following Whole-Body Irradiation			
Mongolian Gerbil	250 KVP	1000	~10
Mouse	200 KVP	640	~10
Mouse (germ-free)	250 KVP	705	—
Rat	250 KVP	714	~12
Dog	1.1 MeV gamma	250	~15
Monkey *"Macaca mulatta"*	250 KVP	600	~14
Rabbit	250 KVP	750	~10
Guinea pig	200 KVP	450	~12
Hamster *Mesocricetus auratus*	200 KVP	610	—
Cricetulus griseus	250 KVP	856	—
Swine	1000 KVP	250	~17
Goat	200 KVP	240	—
Burro	1.1 MeV gamma	255	—
Man	Gamma	300 (?)	~30

Table 1.   LD$_{50/30}$ for   various   species   following   whole—body irradiation.

within the first 30 days following exposure) was related to damage to one of three critical systems; the hemopoietic system following exposures in the middle lethal range, the gastrointestinal syndrome for exposures in the high lethal range and the central nervous system for exposures in the supralethal range.

Of these three radiation syndromes, the hemopoietic continues to receive the most attention since it is the one where therapy may lead to survival of the animal. Nearly 80 years ago Heineke (1905) first showed that the blood forming tissues in rats, rabbits, mice, and guinea pigs reacted strongly, and on the basis of their crude measurements not too dissimilarly, to whole body x-irradiation. Even to this day much of the information available on the effects of ionizing radiation on the hemopoietic system is still descriptive in nature without a clear understanding of mechanisms and their relative importance to the death or survival of the whole body exposed animal. However, there is reason to believe a relationship exists between the time of death and the severe thrombopenia, granulocytopenia and infection often present at the time of death. Similarly, whereas hemorrage is apparent in some species and its pathogenesis has been quite well understood for a number of years (Cronkite et al., 1951, Jackson et al., 1952, Upton, 1955), its role and the accompanying anemia, in mortality is still under discussion.

The difficulty in describing a common clinical response and its relationship to hemopoiesis time parameters and death in various mammals has been discussed in detail by Fliedner (1969) and is well illustrated in Figures 1 and 2. It is apparent that the syndrome developing in man at 25 to 35 days was evident in most other animals at 14 to 21 days. In guinea pigs, mice and rabbits receiving LD_{50} exposures, granulocytopenia was much more pronounced early after exposure and was actually beginning to recover when thrombocytopenia reached maximum levels. The anemia, is of less consequence in humans but increases in importance in monkeys, dogs and guinea pigs, while being most important in mice and rats. It is also apparent that the primary injury leading to the ultimate death of the individual animal in the midlethal dose range is due to injury to the blood precursor cells located for the most part in the bone marrow. The histopathology of such changes has been described by a number of authors and is summarized in considerable detail by Bond et al. (1965). It should also be noted that whereas the changes seen in the mammalian marrow are in general quite similar, the sequence of events differs radically in different species and the relative damage from a given dose of radiation is highly species dependent, with the damage being more related to species than to the absolute radiation dose. An exposure which will virtually deplete the bone marrow of a dog within a few days, may have only minor effects in rodents.

The time course of events leading to death do not differ too significantly from species to species (essentially all deaths occurring before day 25) with the exception of the human where a significant number of deaths may occur between 25 and 60 days. In considering man's relationship to other animals, it appears that he is more similar to swine and dogs in terms of the bone marrow syndrome. In man, both infection and hemorrhage are predominant findings which present clinical problems, whereas although important, anemia is of somewhat less consequence.

In general the larger mammals are more sensitive to the acute effects of ionizing radiation than are the smaller ones, however, injury and recovery generally occur earlier in the smaller species. (Alpen, 1967.)

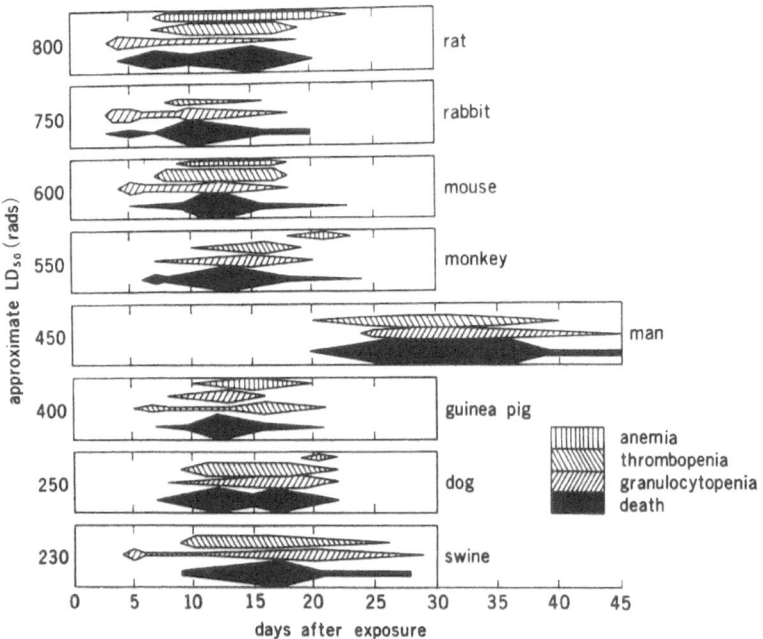

Figure 1. Correlation of time of death with degree of neutropenia in irradiated animals. LD/50 refers to $LD_{50/30}$ days. (From Fliedner 1969)

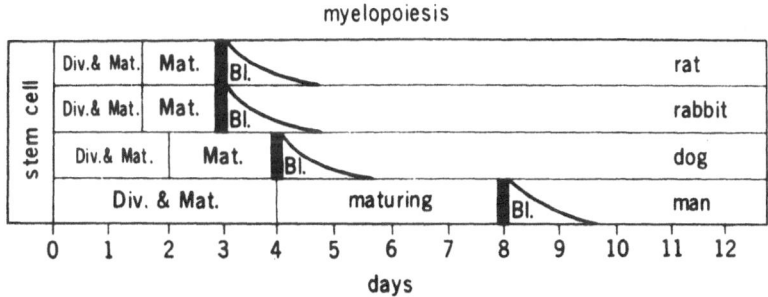

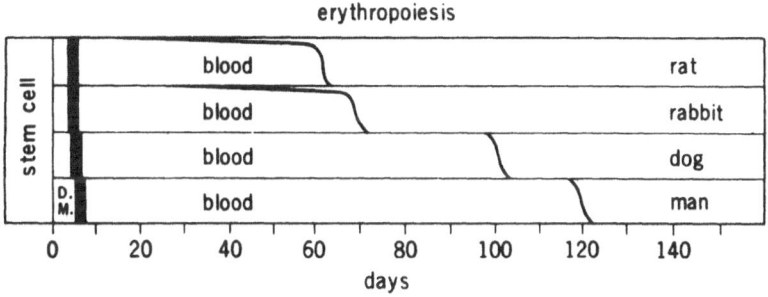

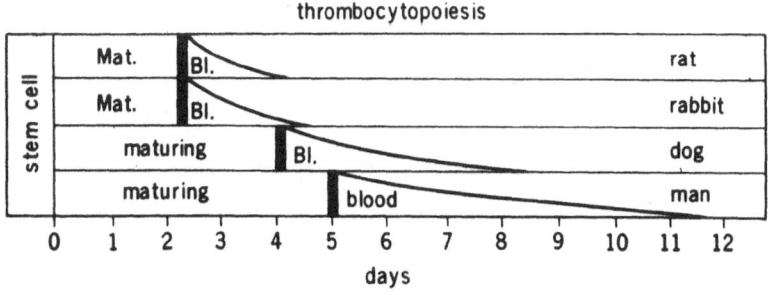

Figure 2.   Summary of estimated time parameters for hemopoiesis in the rat, rabbit, dog, and man.   (Fliedner 1969)

A number of factors may be involved in determining whether or not an irradiated animal can maintain a sufficient number of functional cells to sustain itself during the recovery of the progenitor or stem cell compartment. Some of these factors first described by Patt and Quastler, 1963, are related to the developmental pathway of the functional hematopoietic cells. The importance of individual factors were later defined by Patt, 1968 as follows:

"For various cell compartments, the factors contributing to the relative depletion of the mature functional cells derived from an irradiated steady state population are:

1) stem cell compartment -- the turnover and/or recruitment potential,

2) proliferative compartment -- transit time, number of divisions and amplification potential,

3) maturation compartment -transit time (which probably has little effect), and

4) functional compartment -- the transit or lifetime."

It is perhaps within these characteristics of the cell renewal system that species or strain differences should be investigated for a better understanding of the basis for differences in radiosensitivity.

The "Abortive Rise"

In considering species variability in the hemopoietic radiation syndrome, some consideration should be made of the species variability in the phenomena known as the abortive rise. The abortive rise is that increase in cell numbers which appears to be ubiquitous in irradiated renewal cell systems occurring at various times in various species. Its magnitude appears to be a function of dose, and though apparent in the mature and functional cell pool, it has its origin in an abortive regenerative process that took place earlier in the stem cell compartment. Exact mechanisms involved in the abortive rise have as yet not been clearly defined although several possible causes have been suggested, all of which may have some impact on the phenomenon. The possibilities suggested by Bond (1965) include: "(1) fluctuations in demand, or rate of usage of cells; (2) the stem cell compartment is actually two essentially separate stem cell compartments under normal conditions; (3) temporary failure of feedback or control mechanisms; and most likely; (4) surviving stem cells actually represent two populations of stem cells, one injured and one intact."

In considering this last phenomenon, dying cells are lethally damaged and disappear rapidly from the system, whereas less seriously injured cells will continue to proliferate as evidenced by a rise in number, but result in progeny which die after a few divisions. Key to the ultimate survival of the animal are those cells which either by their more resistant nature or due to their deposition in a more "friendly" environment, survive and lead to the repopulation of the stem cell pool and the survival of the animal. Whereas it is convenient to describe these differences in injured cells as being distinctly different populations, they may well be essentially equivalent cells being irradiated in different stages of the mitotic cycle making them more or less radiosensitive.

Factors Effecting Hemopoietic Radiation Response

The physical and biological factors modifying the hemopoietic response are the definitive subjects of other papers presented in this symposium. Therefore, detailed description of either the physical or biological factors described by other authors will not be attempted except to the extent of brief comments describing factors which may be important in understanding species differences in hemopoietic response to radiation.

The physical factors in terms of dose distribution, bone marrow dose, split dose recovery and dose rate effects have already been described in this symposium (Zoetelief, Broerse, Scott, Schnanzalar, Ainsworth). However, there are two additional factors which may be important in special cases involving the hematopoietic syndrome, and thus deserve some comment. These factors are partial body and nonuniform exposure.

Partial Body Exposure and Shielding effects

While partial body exposure of limited areas or high dose whole body exposure may lead to death through failure of specific organ systems (gut exposure -- gastrointestinal syndrome and brain exposure -- central nervous system syndrome) variations in the hematopoietic syndrome and related death of the animal may be seen in animals where something less than a whole body exposure is given. The earliest instance of a protective influence from shielding a portion of the hemopoietic system was reported by Jacobson et al., 1949, in which shielding the exteriorized spleen increased the $LD_{50/28}$ from 550 R to 975 R in mice. It became apparent that shielding of sufficient hemopoietic stem cells will result in protection of some animals manifested by changes in the $LD_{50/30}$ without a significant modification in the mode or time of death. Such exposure should not be confused with entire upper or lower body exposure where the death may be accounted for by injury to systems other than the hemopoietic. More typical of the situation under discussion are the changes in the $LD_{50/30}$ caused by shielding small areas of the intact animal such as a single leg or the tail in mice. (Robinson, 1965; Carsten, 1968, 1969.)

The accepted explanation for the protective effect of such shielding is that sparing of the shielded stem cells allows reseeding of areas devoid of stem cells due to the radiation exposure. The efficiency of this autorepopulation as compared with external marrow transfusion of an equivalent number of stem cells has been considered by several investigators. In work by Carsten and Cronkite (1971) one group of mice received whole body x-ray exposures with one leg shielded, thus allowing the shielded leg to reseed the exposed animal. A second group of animals receiving a similar exposure had the shielded leg amputated immediately after exposure and its marrow contents totally harvested by a grinding technique (Bond and Stoner 1963) and the marrow reinjected into the same animal. The use of the quanitative grinding technique assured that all shielded cells were reinjected i.v. as opposed to similar studies by other investigators in which only shaft marrow was reinfused. Flushing of the shaft results in harvest of only approximately 70% of the leg bones CFUs' (Carsten, unpublished data).

Results of the above studies indicated that autorepopulation of the animals was more efficient than autotransplant, suggesting that attempts at aiding a partially shielded radiation accident victim to reseed his own marrow from shielded areas might not be of clinical value.

Age of Animal

The age of exposed animals is an important factor in determining their radiosensitivity. In most cases, the immature animal is more radiosensitive, while young adults tend to be more resistant and older animals increase in sensitivity with age. Ignoring prenatal exposure, the maximum sensitivity for rats occurs during the first day where an $LD_{50}/30$ of approximately 225 rads is apparent. In contrast, newborn mice exhibit a certain degree of radioresistance which rapidly disappears with their sensitivity passing through a maximum value at approximately 3 to 4 weeks of age. The studies in rats indicate acute pathologic changes in weanlings and adults to be similar, suggestive of the same mechanism of death with a greater radiosensitivity in the tissues of the young. Casarett (1968) has suggested that the increased sensitivity may be related to the higher mitotic rate of most tissues in the young rapidly growing rats as compared with adults, whereas the extreme sensitivity of the very young rat might be related to the inability of such animals to respond to stress prior to the establishment of the hypothalamic-pituitary-adrenal system.

While the system of most interest in the midlethal range is the hemopoietic, the relative contribution of marrow damage and intestinal injury to death in the LD_{50} range is somewhat age and species dependent. Yuhas and Storer (1967) examined the effect of age on the hematopoietic syndrome in C57BL/6J mice between the ages of 3 and 24 months. They found that resistance to the hemopoietic syndrome increased to a maximum at 17 to 19 months of age as opposed to a decrease in resistance for the gastrointestinal syndrome from 3 months onward. They related the resistance to marrow death in the older animals to an increased number of stem cells in the femoral marrow of the aging mouse, leading to greater numbers of surviving stem cells, thus allowing effective repopulation of the marrow pool following exposure.

Species differences in gastrointestinal response are also evident with the rat showing a greater intestinal sensitivity than either the mouse or the dog (Bond et al., 1965).

Strain Variability

In addition to variation in radiosensitivity between species, considerable variation in sensitivity is noted between various animal strains within species. In 1954 Reinhard et al. observed differences in the relative radiosensitivity of DBA, Marsh, C57BL and C3H mice on the basis of whole body including head, head only or body only x-ray exposures. The $LD_{50}/30$ for whole body, including head exposures, varied from a low of 492 R to 570 R, whereas for head only exposure, the variation was from 500 R to 1443 R, and for body only 735 R to 1265 R. They explained the difference in head sensitivity on the basis of differing pituitary sensitivity leading in turn to corticosteroid insufficiency which might be a contributing factor to the death of the animals. In 1956 Kohn and Kallman investigated the x-ray sensitivity of 4 inbred strains and 2 hybrid strains of mice ranging in age from 91 to 231 days. They found an $LD_{50}/28$ of 665 R for C3H mice, 632 R for A/HE's, 618 R for C57BL and 541 R for BALB/c. A BALB/c A/He cross gave progeny with an $LD_{50}/28$ of approximately 650 R suggesting that the lower LD_{50} of the BALB/c strain was an expression of a recessive genetic factor. A subsequent study by these authors (1957) indicated that all strains showed the same recovery as measured by a two-exposure technique, indicating that the amount of irreversible injury was equivalent in all strains.

Gowen et al. (1943, 1956) and Stadler (1957) examined in some detail the contributions to survival made by body cells of genetically different strains of mice following x-irradiation. The LD_{50} for the strains tested were S,537 R; Q,528 R; Z,522 R; K,481 R and Ba,438 R. Their results were not unlike those of Henshaw (1944) in which he noted that C_3H mice were more sensitive than LAF_1 mice to whole body radiation as measured by both survival and changes in the blood picture.

In a series of studies Grahn and Hamilton (1957) and Grahn (1958) investigated the genetic variation in inbred mouse strains and the expression of radiosensitivity of mice derived from a cross between radiosensitive and radioresistant strains. Their findings included the following: (1) The $LD_{50/30}$ for single whole body x-ray exposure for the inbred strains varied from 500 R to 630 R, (2) There was a positive relationship between the dosage-mortality slope and the LD_{50} value between stains indicating a basic within-strain phenotypic variance, which is positively correlated with susceptibility, (3) Age was a major variable in all strains with radioresistance increasing progressively between 60 and 110 days, (4) Parity and litter size showed minor or inconsistent effects, (5) No significant sex differences were noted in either the dosage-mortality curve slopes or the $LD_{50/30}$ values, (6) The time and rate of recovery of the hemopoietic system are the major physiological variables in the expression of genetic differences in the acute radiation response, (7) The acute lethal response to whole body x-irradiation of F1, F2 and F3 generations from parent resistant and sensitive strains are shown to manifest both nonadditive and additive genetic effects. The variance of sensitivity measured by the dosage-mortality slope is additive, the $LD_{50/30}$ dose is nonadditive, (8) Radiosensitivity is associated to some extent with the albino gene, although the data do not permit discrimination between pleiotropism or linkage as the basis of this association, (9) In the F2 generation, the genetic component of variance (heritability) accounts for about 55% of the variation in radiation sensitivity, and most importantly for the purpose of this presentation, (10). It is postulated that the time and rate of recovery of the hemopoietic system are the major physiological variables in the expression of genetic differences in the acute radiation response.

In subsequent studies, Frölén et al. (1961) examined the importance of genetic background for determining radiosensitivity in an albino strain having an $LD_{50/30}$ value for whole body x-irradiation of 446 R and a CBA strain having a 748 R value. The F1 and F2 generations from a cross between these strains gave a value of 670 R. In a subsequent comparison between C3H's and CBA's showing 668 R and 748 R LD_{50}'s, respectively, the F1 and F2 generations showed values of 725 R and 745 R. These results indicate that resistance cannot be ascribed soley to the action of dominant genes. In other studies by Kondo et al. (1969) using 10 inbred mouse stains, they found a variability for the whole body $LD_{50/30}$ ranging from 547 R to 790 R. In trying to determine what factors may be responsible for the difference in radiation sensitivity between C57BL and CF1 mice, Tsuchiya et al. (1969) measured erythropoietic and stem cell population in both strains. With these techniques they separated out the difference between the degree of injury and the recovery ability of the erythropoietic tissue as measured by ^{59}Fe incorporation and by "exo- and auto-repopulating methods." Their results indicated that the nucleated cells of the leg bone marrow in exposed mice have similar radiosensitivity and proliferative rates, while at the same time it appears that the more radioresistant animals contain more nucleated and stem cells than do the sensitive strains. The observation of a larger stem cell pool, thus leading to the survival of a greater number of cells in an irradiated animal and hence greater survival probability is consistent with the observation by Lajtha et al. (1962) that the size of the stem cell pool is important in determining radiosensitivity. An increased number of stem cells in older animals has also been used to explain the sometimes observed greater radioresistance of older animals as previously noted in this paper.

Increasing number of CFUs through surgical stress has also been shown to increase survival differentially between two Mouse strains having differing autoimmune characteristics (Pachciarz and Teague, 1975).

While instances of differences in radiosensitivity of the hematopoietic system, particularly in mice, are many, a similar difference in radiosensitivit of the gastrointestinal tract has been shown in two strains of rats. Avetisov (1978) found that while the whole body radiosensitivity of Wistar and mongrol rats was equivalent, when abdominally exposed the Wistar rats were significantly more radiosensitive, indicating relative differential radiosensitivity for different organs within the same and different strains.

Cellular Versus Species Radiosensitivity

The temptation exists to attempt a correlation between the shape of the hemopoietic stem cell survival curve and the shape of the whole animal survival curve. Robinson (1969) has analyzed, in terms of cellular parameters, interanimal variations of hemopoietic radioresistance. While his work deals more specifically with sensitivity at the cellular level, a brief examination of his work will lead to cognizance of the problems involved in explaining variation in radiation response at the whole animal level. Robinson formulated a model of acute mammalian hemopoietic radiation mortality relating the dose survival curve of a population of animals with their stem cell survival curve. He assumed that survival of the individual is predicated on maintaining a certain threshold number of effective mature cells which may be specified by a threshold function present at a specific time after irradiation. In addition, he specifies a random variable "effective proliferation factor" describing the proliferation initiated per stem cell. Then, with the further assumption that survival of stem cells obeys Poisson statistics, animal survival probability at any given dose is thus uniquely determined. This probability was shown to give a nearly normal S-shaped dose survival curve with the mean survival dose and width of the curve related to several stem cell parameters. The width of the curve depending principally on randomness in the number of stem cells surviving and the effective proliferation per stem cell as well as interanimal variation of radiosensitivity, which in turn may be dependent upon several interanimal parameters. From Robinson's work, it is apparent that the shape of the mamma- lian dose survival curve is not the same as that for cellular survival curves. Thus, even with the possibility of obtaining "D_0" and "n" values for mammalian survival curves it does not appear that these parameters, which work well for describing cellular populations, would be meaningful parameters for characterizing mamallian resistance, even within one species such as the mouse where the CFUs technique of Till and McCulloch (1961) allows the measurement of a stem cell population. Information on variations in hemopoietic tissue radiosensitivity among species does not supply information which would explain the differences in whole animal radiation sensitivity as measured by the $LD_{50}/_{30}$, however the D_0 continues to be a reasonable measurement for whole animal sensitivity.

A principle conclusion of Robinson is that the steepness of the animal dose survival curve sets an upper limit on the possible values of the interanimal variation of the stem cell inverse slope parameter, D_0.

Additional Comments on Strain Differences

A number of studies have investigated the relationship of survival kinetics for endogenous colony forming units and how this parameter may relate to survival of the whole animal. Till and McCulloch (1964), Smith et al. (1966), and Yuhas and Storer (1967) found a correlation between CFUS kinetics and survival, whereas in other studies, some by the same investigators, a similar correlation was not apparent: Smith et al. (1967), Brecher et al. (1967), Fred et al. (1968) and Yuhas and Storer (1969).

Of particular interest regarding strain variations is the paper by Yuhas and Storer (1969). Using 9 strains of inbred mice they observed that the $LD_{50/30}$'s varied from 616 R ± 12.8 R to 777 ± 7.5 R for acute whole body exposures. When the same strains received 100 R per day exposures, the mean survival time ranged from 17.2 ± 0.5 days to 26.4 ± 0.7 days. When the radiation sensitivity of the endogenous colony forming ability of these same strains was measured, the D_0 was found to vary from 57.1 ± 4.0 R to 83.8 ± 7.3 R. These results indicated that there was no correlation between the whole animal survival and the survival of endogenous spleen colony forming cells. These studies tend to emphasize the complexity of the many factors which enter into survival of the animal in the LD_{50} range.

Further evidence for dissociation of the sensitivity of colony forming cells and the survival of the whole animal is evident from the work of Krebs and Jones (1972). The $LD_{50/30}$ and survival of bone marrow colony forming cells were measured in mice receiving ^{60}Co gamma exposures at either 1750 R per hour or 190 R per hour. The $LD_{50/30}$ was 873 R at 1750 R per hour and 1359 R at 190 R per hour. The D_0 values were 90.1 R and 92.9 R, respectively, indicating that large differences in LD_{50} were not associated with corresponding differences in response of the bone marrow colony forming cells.

A further complicating factor in considering the mechanisms involved in hematopoietic injury and survival of the animal relates to possible differences in radiosensitivity of hemopoietic precursor cells depending upon their source. To date, the spleen colony forming assay remains as the most acceptable method for measuring what is usually considered the pluripotent stem cell. Although the CFUs may be obtained from a number of tissues including the bone marrow, adult spleen, fetal liver, peritoneal fluid, and peripheral blood, there is no unquestionable evidence that these are the same cells or that they might supply equal regenerative ability in the exposed animal and therefore equal protection. To the contrary, Siminovitch et al. (1965) compared the radiation survival curves for colony forming cells derived from fetal liver, spleen and adult femoral marrow. They found D_0 values and extrapolation numbers of 95 ± 9 rads, 1.50 ± 0.54 for adult bone marrow; 90 ± 16 rads for adult spleen, 0.80 ± 0.46 and 146 ± 26 rads, 1.08 ± 0.50 for fetal liver. To determine whether these differences in sensitivity between cell types were heritable differences, they compared the colony forming cells from various sources but growing under identical conditions in the irradiated hosts. Cells from bone marrow, fetal liver and spleen were injected into irradiated animals and allowed to proliferate for 14 days, after which time cells were harvested from the recipient spleen or femoral marrow and tested for colony forming efficiencies and radiation sensitivity. At that time, the cells showed a uniform but increased radiation sensitivity; D_0 of 69 ± 12 R for the marrow cells, 74 ± 15 R for the spleen cells and 80 ± 16 R for the fetal liver derived cells. These findings indicate that attempts at a simplified theory of animal survival depending upon total stem cells regardless of their origin is not reasonable since the radiation sensitivity may vary significantly depending upon the previous history of the cells.

These authors also determined that the early radiation sensitivity of colony forming cells tended to be a reversible effect with a return to normal radiosensitivity seen after a period of several months. While not defined in nature, these changes may well be related to the so-called reparable portion of radiation injury.

Effect of Dose Rate, Oxygen, Temperature and Hibernation

Effects of dose rate on the hemopoietic syndrome in large animals will be discussed during this symposium by Ainsworth. However, it should be pointed out that effects similar to those found in large animals are seen in mice as well. Neal (1960) demonstrated that the $LD_{50/30}$ for mice could be increased from 788 R to 1097 R by lengthening the duration of whole body x-ray exposure from 1 minute to 8 hours. Similar findings have been demonstrated for pulsed or fractionated exposures. The increase in $LD_{50/30}$ is apparently due to a reduction in the "effective" dose and not due to a change in the character of injury or the mode of death. For a further discussion of dose rate effects, see Caserett (1968), pages 244–249, and the previous cited paper by Yuhas and Stover (1969).

STUDIES AT BROOKHAVEN NATIONAL LABORATORY

Over the last approximately 30 years a number of studies have been carried out in the Medical and Biology Departments at Brookhaven National Laboratory aimed at gaining a better understanding of the factors involved in the acute hematopoietic radiation syndrome. The following paragraphs will contain brief descriptions of some of these studies not already referred to in the previous discussion.

Nonuniform Exposures

While whole body and partial body exposure studies are interesting and informative concerning the overall damage to the hemopoietic system and for the prediction of mortality following mid-lethal exposures, in the human situation involving nuclear weapons or accidents, the exposure may well be more of a nonuniform nature. The question of whether or not the classical "stem cell survival model" stating that survival of the animal depends on a critical surviving fraction of stem cells applies for uniform and nonuniform exposure requires testing and verification. If the stem cell distribution in various parts of the body, the radiation doses to these parts, and the dose survival curve for stem cells are known, it seems reasonable that the survival for nonuniform exposed animals could be calculated in the same way that is done for the whole body or partial body exposed animal. Bond and Robinson (1967) tested this hypothesis on the basis of evaluating the results of other investigators work involving bilateral and unilateral exposures of dogs and swine. (Ainsworth et al. 1964, Tullis et al. 1949, Tullis et al. 1950). Because at that time distribution of active marrow was unknown in these animals, the authors applied the information available for man (Atkinson

1963). From evaluation of available those data they developed a concept of the distribution effectiveness factor (DEF) which is defined as the quotient of the average nonuniform dose divided into the equivalent (on the basis of the model) uniform dose; thus:

$$D_{EF} = \frac{\text{equivalent uniform dose.}}{\text{average uniform dose.}}$$

This model predicts less efficiency for nonuniform doses; therefore, the DEF is less than 1.0.

To further investigate the question of nonuniform exposures, a series of studies were undertaken to measure the distribution of active bone marrow and the regional absorbed dose to areas of interest in mice receiving nonuniform gamma exposures.

The active bone marrow distribution and related stem cell content were determined by established radioisotope and stem cell methodologies. Bone marrow distribution was determined by injecting mice with radioiron ^{59}Fe and then determining the amount of activity present at the end of 24 hours in 1 cm. transverse segments of mice that were anesthetized, placed in the exact position used for irradiation, frozen in liquid nitrogen and sectioned. The distribution of stem cells was determined throughout the skeletal system by the spleen colony assay (Till and McCulloch, 1961) on cells obtained using the quantitative grinding technique (Stoner and Bond, 1963). For results of these determinations see Taketa 1970. Nonuniform exposures were carried out using a spoked wheel arrangement around a central ^{137}Cs source (Figure 3). Animals placed with either the head or tail end near the source were given a nonuniform exposure using either a 400 Curie or a 1,600 Curie source. The difference in source size allowed for exposures at the same dose rate at different distances from the source. At greater distances the nonuniformity was less due to the diminishing contribution of the inverse square law, thus allowing comparison of 2 degrees of nonuniformity. Comparison of nonuniform exposure effects to those from uniform exposures were made by exposing mice bilaterally around the circumference of a wheel with the animals being reversed midway through the exposure to ensure uniformity of dose within the animal. Depth dose distribution was established in the irradiated animals by lithium flouride thermoluminescent dosimeters implanted at 1 cm. intervals along the spinal axis of a frozen mouse carcass. In Figure 4 is shown the depth dose distribution using the 400 and 1600 Curie sources as well as the bone marrow distribution as measured by the radioiron uptake. Superimposed in this figure is seen an x-ray of a mouse in the irradiation apparatus giving an indication of relative bone positions. $LD_{50/30}$ determinations using the 1,600 Curie source gave values for head-on irradiation of 988 R, tail-on 981 R and for uniform exposure 975 R. Determinations using the smaller source did not show the same similarity. The radioiron distribution indicated a bipeaked pattern nearly symmetrical around the midpoint of the animal. The two peaks are apparently due to the greater marrow content of the upper and lower legs. To consider the hypothesis presented by Bond (1969), it would be necessary to make an exact summation or integration using the marrow distribution, the depth dose distribution and the dose survival curve for individual marrow cells. However, since the marrow distribution to a first approximation is symmetrical around the midpoint, and since the depth dose curve falls off with the same pattern when measured with either end of the animal near the source, a reasonable examination of the hypothesis can be made by a simple comparison of the $LD_{50/30}$ values as specified above. The close agreement in those values

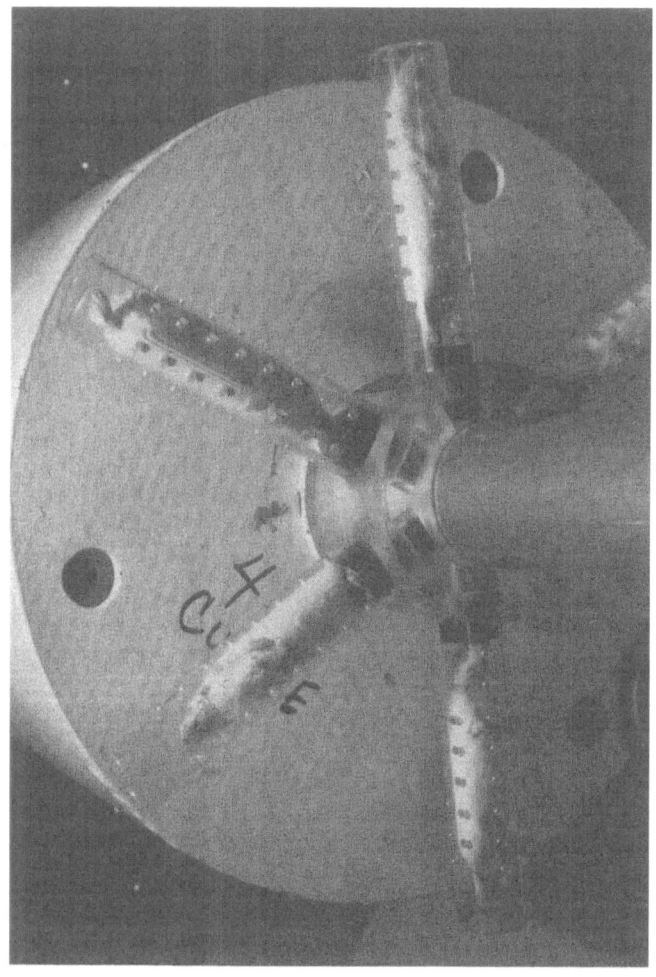

Figure 3. Apparatus for nonuniform irradiation of mice showing spoke-
wheeled arrangement with source located in central tube.
Note: Mice ar alternately placed with head or rear towards
source.

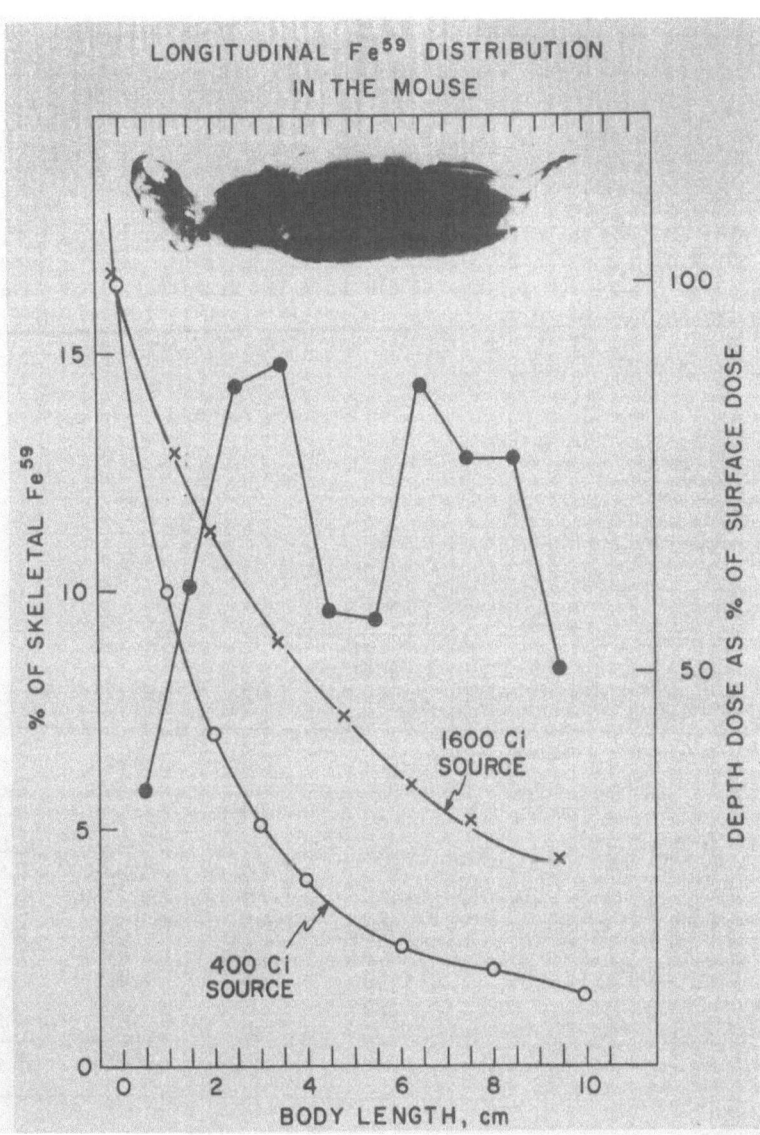

Figure 4. Depth dose distribution and ^{59}Fe distribution in mice.
X – depth dose from 1600 Ci source
O – depth dose from 400 Ci source
● – ^{59}Fe distribution in 1 centimeter body segments..

indicated that for nonuniform exposures when the ratio of the extremes of dose is not too great, the Bond hypothesis probably holds true.

Variations in $LD_{50/30}$ for the HS/BNL Mouse

It is well established that different mouse and rat strains show variation in radiosensitivity when examined over long periods of time. The sensitivity of the Hale-Stoner/BNL mouse has been tested for changes in whole body 250 kVp x-ray radiosensitivity for a period of approximately 15 years. The changes in $LD_{50/30}$ are shown in Table 2.

The $LD_{50/30}$ for determinations on male animals indicated a mean value of 621 R with a range of 573-662. Comparable values for the females were: $LD_{50/30}$, 665 R with a range of 618 to 713. Note that the values for regular water as opposed to acid water indicated slightly lower LD_{50}'s. The use of acid water was instituted when it was discovered that the colony had become infected with pseudomonas.

Variation in $LD_{50/30}$ for HS/BNL Mice
1969 — 1978

Date	Age (wks.)	Sex	Water	Total Animals	$LD_{50/30}$	95% C.I.	s.d.
8/69	8	M	R*	543	606	593-620	6.9
11/70	8	M	A**	250	662	648-675	7.0
7/70	8	M	A	80	615	599-630	7.8
10/71	8-10	F	R	300	612	579-646	16.9
1/73	8-10	M	A	250	619	608-630	5.6
1/75	10	F	A	138	713	688-738	12.8
3/75	8-10	M	A	490	654	646-662	4.0
8/76	10-12	M	R	420	660	653-667	3.6
3/77	10-12	M	A	240	605	584-626	10.6
8/78	8-12	F	A	480	618	605-631	6.6
8/78	8-12	M	A	120	586	541-631	23.0
11/78	8-12	M	A	299	573	535-611	19.4

*Tap water
**Acidified water; pH=2.4

Table 2.   Variation in $LD_{50/30}$ for HS/BNL mice (1969-1978).

During this time, the bone marrow stem cell radiosensitivity was also determined using the Till and McCullough (1961) in vivo technique. No large variations in radiosensitivity were noted during the times when the colony exhibited extremes in $LD_{50/30}$ values. On that basis, it is assumed that the minor variations in $LD_{50/30}$'s were not related to inherent differences in stem cell population but to other factors affecting the colony such as bacterial infection, normal seasonal variations, etc. The mean survivial times of animals dying within the 30 day observation period were 11.3 days for female animals and 13.4 days for male animals. The somewhat shorter survival time for the female animals can be attributed to a rather large incidence of death on the 7th day in one experiment. This took place in a group of animals which were found to have a pseudomonas infection. If those animals are eliminated, the mean survival time for females is essentially equivalent to the male animals.

It might be noted that during one short period our animal colony became infested with mites. While the presence of these mites caused small skin lesions in the irradiated and unirradiated animals, there was no effect on their radiosensitivity during this brief period of infestation.

Our observations concerning variaion in $LD_{50/30}$ do not differ significantly in magnitude with those of Udupa et al. (1974), who followed a strain of rats over a 20-year period. They observed LD_{50}'s ranging from 710 to 950 R with a mean of 801 R. They explain the variations on the basis of general health of the colony. The advent of infections was seen to reduce the $LD_{50/30}$ somewhat, while long term exposure of the colony to infection increases the $LD_{50/30}$ dose level slightly and gave some protection against hemopoietic damage. One might hypothesize that the increased resistance with long-term infections was due to the stimulation of the stem cell pool, resulting in an expansion which in turn would allow for a greater surviving member of stem cells following radiation, thus allowing survival of a greater number of animals.

RBE Studies on Hemopoietic Cells

There is continuing interest in defining precise relationships between linear-energy transfer (LET) and biological effect relationships for the hemopoietic system. Reasons for this include: (1) renewed interest in the therapeutic use of high LET radiations, (2) knowledge of the LET is essential to the formulation of any theory defining basic mechanisms in radiobiology and (3) for radiation protection or health physics purposes, LET versus effect relationships are essential in establishing radiation protection standards. In the Brookhaven studies, radiations investigated included 250 kVp x-rays, monoenergenic neutrons of discrete energies ranging from 0.43 MeV to 13.4 MeV, gamma rays from [182]Ta as well as reactor and [252]Cf fission neutrons. Exposures ranged from 20 to 200 rads. Using the 250 kVp x-rays as a standard and exogenous CFUS killing as the effect, the RBE for monoenergenic neutrons ranges from 0.85 for 13.4 MeV neutrons to 2.8 for 1.0 and 0.43 MeV neutrons. Fission neutrons from the reactor delivered at 20 R per minute gave an RBE of 1.58. [252]Cf neutrons delivered at 0.18 R per minute gave an RBE of 1.59. The calculated D_0 for the 250 kVp x-rays was 80.14 ± 2.17 R for exposure at 120 R per minute. For further details of this study, see Carsten et al. (1976).

The RBE of different energy neutrons on human bone marrow cells was also determined using both in vivo diffusion chamber (DC) techniques and in vitro techniques. Based on the survival of proliferative granulocytes, in (DC) on day 13 of culture the D_0 value for 250 kVp x-rays was found to be 80 R as compared to 117 R using in vitro techniques. The RBE values, which dropped with increasing energy levels of monoenergetic neutrons, ranged from 3.7 at 0.44 MeV to 1.6 at 15 MeV in (DC), with comparable values for in vitro determinations of 4.1 and 1.6. Fission neutrons gave values of 2.6 for (DC) culture and 2.4 for in vitro culture. It should be noted that although the human and the mouse exhibit very different $LD_{50/30}$ values, the D_0 values for the bone marrow progenitor cells are quite similar. For further information see Boyum et al. (1978).

SUMMARY

It is apparent from a rather detailed examination of the literature that after 80 years of exposing numerable mammalian species to ionizing radiation there are still many unanswered questions concerning the basis for differences in species radiosensitivity. Rather than to reiterate the comments already made in the body of this paper, I will instead present what is basically a listing of unanswered questions or subjects requiring further investigation which might supply useful information for understanding the basis for differences in species radiosensitivity. To phrase it another way, "what don't we know that might be important?"

1. Dosimetry remains an important question. In considering mortality in the mid-lethal range, we must know more precisely the dose distribution at the whole body level and perhaps even more so at the hemopoietic stem cell level. Consideration should be made that the dose to marrow cells at bone-soft tissue interfaces may be quite different from that for cells surrounded by soft tissue.

2. Hematopoietic stem cell distribution throughout the body of different species and its change with age are important factors in understanding mortality in the $LD_{50/30}$ range, once the dosimetry question is answered.

3. A better understanding of the importance of stromal or hematopoietic microenvironmental factors in defining radiosensitivity is necessary. More information is needed concerning both the radiosensitivity and repair capabilities of stromal tissues which support hemopoietic stem cell growth.

4. Importance of organ system interactions following the stress of irradiation deserves some attention. Mention is made in the previously cited literature concerning radiation induced stress and the importance of hormonal factors, however a clear delineation of these factors has not been made.

5. The role of immune competence has not been sufficiently defined in enough species to determine its place in the survival of the exposed animal.

6. Can anything be learned from species variation in the "abortive rise" phenomenon concerning the importance of injured cells and their ability to modify survival of the animal?

7. Can we learn anything more from split dose and variable dose rate determinations?

8. Can we learn anything more from shielding studies and non-uniform exposures?

9. The importance of DNA repair mechanisms and possible differences in various species should be further investigated to determine whether or not these factors may account for some of the differences in radiationsensitivity. In terms of repair, particular attention might be given to the importance of DNA double strand breaks and the survival of the stem cell and thus the whole animal.

10. Related to the previous statement, one is led to believe that a closer examination of other biochemical differences in the hematopoietic stem cells of various species may be informative.

11. To date the majority of information about hematopoietic stem cells is on the mouse. This is due primarily to the ability to accurately measure its marrow stem cell content using the spleen colony forming assay and economic factors related to use of smaller animals. However, for a comparison to other species, it becomes apparent that we must attempt to make determinations of other species stem cell radiosensitivity similar to those in mice. This implies the use of other techniques to determine radiosensitivity of stem cells and its variation with cycle time, etc. Development of such techniques deserve further attention.

It is assumed that many of the items touched upon above will be discussed in great detail by other participants in this workshop and it is thus expected that perhaps answers to some of the questions will be available or at least a concensus concerning the importance of these factors will be summarized by the editors of the proceedings.

ACKNOWLEDGMENTS

Many individuals contributed not only their time and effort to the performance of studies described in this paper but also in several instances contributed their own experimental results and interpretations of data. Among those contributing significant amounts of original information are Drs. V. P. Bond, E. P. Cronkite, C. V. Robinson and R. Stoner. All of these deserve sincere thanks for their generosity in this respect. Leigh Philips, who has over the years contributed much in advice and effort concerning radiation dosimetry deserves special thanks. I would also like to acknowledge the excellent technical help of L. Cook, J. Bullis, J. Cassidy and A. Gremillion, who spent many hours in the laboratory assisting in the studies reported. Finally, I would like to thank D. Pion, Linda Wasson and the Word Processing Center for their efforts in preparing this manuscript. Work supported by the U.S. Department of Energy under Contract No. DE-AC02-76CH00016.

REFERENCES

Abrams, H.L. Influence of age, body weight and sex on susceptibility of mice to lethal effects of x-radiation. Proc. Soc. Exp. Biol. Med. 76:729-732, 1951.

Ainsworth, E.J., Leong, G.F., Kendall, K., and Alpen, E.L. Comparative lethality responses of neutron and x-irradiated dogs: Influence of dose rate and exposure aspect. U.S. Navy Radiological Defense Laboratory Report USNRDL-TR-787 (Oct. 6, 1964).

Ainsworth, E.J., Leong, G.F., Kendall, K., and Alpen, E.L. Comparative lethality responses of neutron- and x-irradiated dogs: Influence of dose rate and exposure aspect. Radiation Res. 26:32-43, 1965.

Al-Hilli, F. and Wright, E.A. The effects of changes in the environmental temperature on the growth of bone in the mouse. Radiological and morphological study. Br. J. Exp. Path. 64:43-50, 1983.

Altus, M.S., Bernstein, S.E., Russell, E.S., Carsten, A.L., and Upton, A.C. Defect extrinsic to stem cells in spleens of steel anemic mice. Proceedings of the Society for Experimental Biology and Medicine 138:985-988, 1971.

Atkinson, H.R. Bone marrow distribution as a factor in estimating radiation to the blood-forming organs; A survey of present knowledge. J. College Radiolo. Australasia 6:149-154, 1963.

Avetisov, G.M., Zharkova, G.P., and Zaitseva, R.N. Comparative radio-sensitivity of Wistar and mongrel rats to nonuniform radiation. Radiobiology, Vol. XVIII, 70-76, 1978.

Bond, V.P. Radiation mortality in different mammalian species. In: Comparative Cellular and Species Radiosensitivity. Eds. V.P. Bond and T. Sugahara, Igaku Shoin Ltd. Tokyo, Japan, 1969, pp. 5-19.

Bond, V.P., Fliedner, T.M. and Archambeau, J.O. Effects of radiation on the hemopoietic system: The bone-marrow syndrome. In: Mammalian Radiation Lethality, Chapter 7, pp 159-230, Academic Press, New York, 1965.

Bond, V.P., Fliedner, T.M., and Archambeau, J.O. The abortive rise. In: Mammalian Radiation Lethality. pp 78-83, Academic Press, New York, 1965.

Bond, V.P. and Robinson, C.V. A mortality determinant in nonuniform exposures of the mammal. Radiation Res. 7:265-275, 1967.

Bond, V.P., and Robinson, C.V. Bone-marrow stem-cell survival in the non-uniformly exposed mammal. In: Effects of Ionizing Radiations on the Haematopoietic Tissue, IAEA Panel, May 17-20, Vienna, 1967.

Bond, V..P., Fliedner, T.M., and Archambeau, J.O. A disturbance in cellular kinetics. In: Mammalian Radiation Lethality. Academic Pres, New York, 1965.

Bond, V.P., and Sugahara, T. Comparative cellular and species radiosensitivity. Igaku Shoin Ltd., Tokyo, 1969.

Bøyum, A., Carsten, A.L., Chikkapa, G., Cook, L., Bullis, J., Honikel, L., and Cronkite, E.P. The RBE of different-energy neutrons as determined by human bone-marrow cell-culture techniques. Int. J. Radiat. Biol. 34:201-121, 1978.

Brecher, G., Ansell, J.D., Micklem, H.S., Tjio, J.H., and Cronkite, E.P. Special proliferative sites are not needed for seeding and proliferation of transfused bone marrow cells in normal syngeneic mice. Proc. Nat. Acad. Sci. USA 79:5085-5087, 1982.

Carsten, A.L., and Cronkite, E.P. Comparison of autologous marrow injection to shielding in lethal irradiation of the mouse. Proc. Soc. Exp. Biol. & Med. 137:948-951, 1971.

Carsten, A.L., and Bond, V.P. CFU content of the x-ray exposed and shielded mouse femur. Exptl. Hematology 15:95-103, 1968.

Carsten, A.L., and Bond, V.P. Colony forming units in the bone marrow of partial body irradiated mice. In: Normal and Malignant Cell Growth, Edited by R.J.M. Fry, M.L. Griem, W.H. Kirsten, Springer-Verlag, New York Inc., 1969.

Carsten, A.L., Bond, V.P., and Thompson, K. The RBE of different energy neutrons as measured by the hematopoietic spleen-colony technique. Int. J. Radiat. Biol. 29:65-70, 1976.

Casarett, A.P. Radiation biology. Prentice-Hall Inc., Englewood, New Jersey, 1968.

Chaffey, J.T., and Hellman, S. Differing responses to radiation of murine bone marrow stem cells in relation to the cell cycle. Cancer Res. 31:1613-1615, 1971.

Congdon, C.C., and Lorenz, E. Humoral factor in irradiation protection: Modification of lethal irradiation injury in mice by injection of rat bone marrow. Am. J. Physiol. 176:297-300, 1954.

Cronkite, E.P., Carsten, A.L., and Brecher, G. Hemopoietic stem cell niches, recovery from radiation and bone marrow transfusions. In: Proceedings of the 6th International Congress of Radiation Research, Eds. S. Okada, M. Imamura, T. Terashima, H. Yamaguchi, pp. 649-656, Toppan Printing Co., Ltd., Tokyo, 1979.

Cronkite, E.P., Jackson, D.P., LeRoy, G.V., and Lundie, A.R.T. The present status of the hemorrhagic aspects of radiation injury. Proc. Int. Soc. Hema., May 1951.

Danysz, J. De l'action pathogene des rayons et des emanations emis par le radium sur differents tissus et differents organismes. Compt. Rend. Acad. d. Sci. 136:461-464, 1903.

Fliedner, T.M. A cytokinetic comparison of Hematological consequences of radiation exposure in different mammalian species. In: Comparative Cellular and Species Radiosensitivity. Eds. V.P. Bond and T. Sugahara, Igaku Shoin Ltd. Tokyo, Japan, 1969, pp. 89-101.

Fliedner, T.M., Bond, V.P., and Cronkite, E.P. Structural, cytologic and autoradiographic (H -thymidine) changes in the bone marrow following total body irradiation. Am. J. Pathology Vol. 38:599-623, 1961.

Fliedner, T.M., and Heit, H. Hematopoietic death in conventional and germfree mice. In: Comparative Cellular and Species Radiosensitivity, Eds. V.P. Bond and T. Sugahara, pp 220-232, Igaku Shoin Ltd., Tokyo, Japan, 1969.

Fred, S.S., and Smith, W.W. Radiation sensitivity and proliferative recovery of hemopoietic stem cells in weanling as compared to adult mice. Radiation Res. 32:314-326, 1967.

Frolen, H., Luning, K.G., and Ronnback, C. The effect of x-irradiation on various mouse strains due to their genetic background. Radiation Res. 14: 381-393, 1961.

Glasgow, G.P., Beetham, K.L., and Mill, W.B. Dose rate effects on the survival of normal hematopoietic stem cells of BALB/c mice. Int. J. Rad. Oncology Biol. Phys. 9:557-563, 1983.

Gowen, J.W., and Zelle, M.R. Irradiation effects on genetic resistance of mice to mouse typhoid. J. Infec. Dis. 77:2-5, 1945.

Gowen, J.W., and Zelle, M.R. Irradiation effects on genetic resistance of mice to mouse typhoid. J. Infect. Dis. 77:85-91, 1945.

Grahn, D. Acute radiation response of mice from a cross between radio-sensitive and radioresistant strains. Genetics 43:835-843, 1958.

Grahn, D. Genetic control of physiological processes: The genetics of radiation toxicity in animals. In: Radioisotopes in the Biosphere, Eds. R.S. Caldecott and L.A. Synder, Minneapolis, Minn., 1960.

Grahn, D. Genetic variations in the response of mice to total body x-irradiation. I. Body weight response in six inbred strains. J. Exp. Zool. 125:39-61, 1954.

Grahn, D., and Hamilton, K.F. Genetic variation in the acute lethal response of four inbred mouse strains to whole body x-irradiation. Genetics 40:1189-1198, 1957.

Hagen, C.W., and Sacher, G.A. Effects of total-body x-irradiation on rabbits. I. Mortality after single and paired doses. Biological Effects of External X and Gamma Radiation. Ed. Raymond E. Zirkle, pp 243-264, McGraw Hill, New York, 1954.

Hanks, G.E. In vivo migration of colony-forming units from shielded bone marrow in the irradiated mouse. Nature 203:1393-1394, 1964.

Hanks, G.E., and Ainsworth, E.J. Repopulation of colony-forming units in mice. Nature 215:20-22, 1967.

Hanks, G.E., Page, N.P., Ainsworth, E.J., Leong, G.F., Menkes, C.K., and Alpen, E.L. Acute mortality and recovery studies in sheep irradiated with cobalt-60 gamma rays or 1-Mvp x-rays. Radiation Res. 27:397-405, 1966.

Heit, H., Fliedner, T.M., Fache, I., and Schnell, G. A comparison of radiation-induced bone marrow degeneration in germfree and conventional mice. Radiation Res. 41:163-182, 1970.

Henshaw, P.S. Experimental roentgen injury. II Changes produced with intermediate-range doses and a comparison of the relative susceptibility of different kinds of animals. JNCI Vol. 4, 5:485-501, 1944.

Hieieneke, H. Experimentelle Untersuchunger über die Enwirkung der Röntgenstrahlen auf innere Organe. Mitt. aus den Grenfgebeten der Medizin und Chirurgie, 14:21-94, 1905.

Hightower, D. Woodward, K.T., McLaughlin, M.M. and Hahn F.F. The effect of age, strain, and exposure intensity on the mortality response of neutron-irradiated mice. Radiation Res. 35:369-377, 1968.

Jackson, D.P., Cronkite, E.P., LeRoy, G.V., and Halpern, B. Further studies on the nature of the hemorrhagic state in radiation injury. J. Lab. and Clin. Med. 39:449-461, 1952.

Jacobson, L.O. Hematologic recovery from radiation injury. In: Progress in Hematology, Eds. Grune and Stratton, Vol. I, 311-320, 1956.

Jacobson, L.O., Marks, E.K., and Gaston, E. Effects of total-body x-irradiation on a preexisting induced anemia in rabbits. II. Response of animals with an anemia induced by bleeding. In: Biological Effects of External X and Gamma Radiation. Ed. Raymond E. Zirkle, pp 330-338, McGraw-Hill, New York, 1954.

Jacobson, L.O., Marks, E.K., and Gaston, E.O. Observations on the effect of spleen-shielding and the injection of cell suspensions on survival following irradiation. Presented at the 5th International Congress of Hematology, Paris, France, Sept. 6-12, 1954.

Jacobson, L.O., Marks, E.K., and Gaston, E.O. Observations on the effect of spleen-shielding and the injection of cell suspensions on survival following irradiation. In: Radiobiology Symposium. Eds. Z.M. Bacq, and Peter Alexander, pp 122, Butterworths Scientific Publications, London, 1955.

Jacobson, L.O., Marks, E.K., and Gaston, E.O. Observations on the effect of spleen-shielding and the injection of cell suspensions on survival following irradiation. Proc. Soc. Exp. Biol. Med. 119, 122-126, New York, 1963.

Jacobson, L.O., Marks, E.D., Gaston, E., and Simmons, E.L. Effects of total-body x-irradiation on a preexisting induced anemia in rabbits. I. Response of animals with anemia induced by phenyldrazine. In: Biological Effects of External X and Gamma Radiation. Ed. Raymond E. Zirkle, pp 317-329, McGraw Hill, New York, 1954.

Jacobson, L.O., Marks, E.K., Simmons, E.L, Hagen, C.W., and Zirkle, R.E. Effects of total-body x-irradiation on rabbits. II. Hematological effects. In: Biological Effects of External X and Gamma Radiation. Ed. Raymond E. Zirkle, pp 265-289, McGraw-Hill, New York, 1954.

Jacobsen, L.O., Marks, E.K., Robson, M.J., Gaston, E., and Zirkle, R.E. The effect of spleen protection on mortality following x-irradiation. J. Lab. Clin. Med. 34:1538-1543, 1949.

Jamieson, D., and van den Brenk, H.A.S. Effect of progressive changes in body temperature of rats on tissue oxygen-tensions, in relation to radiosensitivity. Int. J. Rad. Biol. 6:529-540, 1963.

Kaplan, H.S., and Paull, J. Genetic modification of response to spleen shielding in irradiated mice. Proc. Soc. Exp. Biol. Med. 79:670-672, 1952.

Kohn, H.I., and Kallman, R.F. The influence of strain on acute x-ray lethality in the mouse. I. LD_{50} and death rate studies. Radiation Res. 5:309-317, 1956.

Kohn, H.I., and Kallman, R.F. The influence of strain on acute x-ray lethality in the mouse. II. Recovery Rate Studies. Radiation Res. 6:329-338, 1957.

Kondo, K., Nagami, T., and Teramoto, S. Differences in hematopoietic death among inbred strains of mice. In: Comparative Cellular and Species Radiosensitivity, Eds. V.P. Bond and T. Sugahara, Igaku Shoin Ltd., Tokyo, Japan, pp 20-29, 1969.

Koznova, L.B. Effect of radiation dose rate on median lethal dose for mice with development of hemopoietic and enteric syndromes. In: Radiobiology, DOE-tr-4/9, Vol. 18, pp 63-69, No. 3, 1978.

Krebs, J.S., and Jones, D.C. The LD_{50} and the survival of bone-marrow colony-forming cells in mice: Effect of rate of exposure to ionizing radiation. Radiation Res. 51:374-380, 1972.

Lajtha, L.G., Oliver, R., and Gurney, C.W. Kinetic model of a bone-marrow stem-cell population. Brit. J. Haemt. 8:442-460, 1962.

Leong, G.F., Page, N.P., Ainsworth, E.J., and Hanks, G.E. Injury accumulation and recovery in sheep during protracted gamma irradiation. Radiation Res. 7:288-293, 1967,

Leong, G.F., Wisecup, W.G., Grisham, J.W. Effects of divided doses of x-ray on mortality and hematology of small and large domestic animals. Ann. N.Y. Acad. Sci. 114:138-146, 1964.

Lorenz, E., and Congdon, C.C. Modification of lethal irradiation injury in mice by injection of homologous or heterologous bone. J. Natl. Cancer Inst. 14:955-961, 1954.

Lorenz, E., Congdon, C., and Uphoff, D. Modification of acute irradiation injury in mice and guinea-pigs by bone marrow injections. In: Radiology, Ed. Howard P. Doub, Vol. 58, The Radiological Society of North America, January-June 1952, pp. 863-877.

McCulloch, E.A., and Till, J.E. Proliferation of hemopoietic colony-forming cells transplanted into irradiated mice. Radiation Res. 22:383-397, 1964.

McLaughlin, M.M., Dacquesto, M.P., Jacobus, D.P., and Horowitz, R.E. Effects of the germfree state on responses of mice to whole-body irradiation. Radiation Res. 23:33-349, 1964.

Mirand, E.A., Reinhard, M.C., and Goltz, H.L. Protective effect of adrenal steroid administration on irradiated mice. Proc. Soc. Exp. Biol. Med. 81: 397-380, 1952.

Nachtwey, D.S., Ainsworth, E.J., and Leong, G.F. Recovery from radiation injury in swine as evaluated by the split-dose technique. Radiation Res. 31:353-367, 1967.

Neal, F.E. Variation of acute mortality with dose-rate in mice exposed to single large doses of whole-body x-irradiation. Intern. J. Radiation Biol. 2:295-300, 1960.

Nelson, J.M. Radiobiology of the Mongolian Gerbil. Ph. D. Thesis from the University of Michigan, 1969.

Pachciarz, J.A., and Teague, P.O. Different responses of two mouse strains to 650 rads and protection by surgical stress. Proc. Soc. Exp. Biol. and Med. 148:1095-1100, 1975.

Patt, H.M. Cell turnover and mammalian radiosensitivity. Cell Tissue Kinet. 1:81-88, 1968.

Patt, H.M. Species differences in leukocyte restoration after irradiation. In: Comparative Cellular and Species Radiosensitivity, Eds. V.P. Bond and T. Sugahara, pp 112-122, Igaku Shoin Ltd., Tokyo, Japan, 1969.

Patt, H.M., and Maloney, M. A comparison of radiation-induced granulocytopenia in several mammalian species. Radiation Res. 18:231-235, 1963.

Patt, H.M., and Maloney, M.A. The $bg^J/bg^J:W/W^V$ Bone marrow chimera: A model for studying stem cell regulation. Blood Cells 4:27-35, 1978.

Pettersen, E.O., Boyum, A., and Laane, B.F.M. X-ray inactivation of murine bone marrow cells as measured by the spleen colony assay and the diffusion chamber technique. Radiation Res. 58:409-416, 1974.

Reinhard, M.C., Mirand, E.A., Goltz, H.L., and Hoffman, J.G. Mouse-strain differences in response to radiation. Proc. Soc. Exp. Biol. Med. 85:307-370, 1959.

Riopelle, A.J., Ades, H.W., and Morgan, Jr., F.E. Peripheral Blood of the x-irradiated rhesus monkey. Radiation Res. 7:581-590, 1957.

Robinson, C.V. Analysis in terms of cellular parameters of interanimal variation of hemopoietic radioresistance. In: Comparative Cellular and Species Radiosensitivity. Eds. V.P. Bond, and T. Sugahara, Igaku Shoin Ltd. Tokyo, Japan, 1969, pp. 211-219.

Robinson, C.V. Decrease in numbers of mouse spleen nodules with time post-irradiation. Proc. Soc. Exp. Biol. Med. 124, January-April, New York, 1967, pp. 118-122.

Robinson, C.V. Relationship between animal and stem cell dose-survival curves. Radiation Res. 35:318-344, 1968.

Robinson, C.V., Commerford, S.L., and Bateman, J.L. Evidence for the presence of stem cells in the tail of the mouse. Proc. Soc. Exp. Biol. Med. Vol. 119, pp. 222-269, New York, 1965.

Robinson, C.V., Commerford, S.L., and Bateman, J.L. Evidence for the presence of stem cells in the tail of the mouse. Proc. Soc. Exp. Biol. Med. Vol. 124, New York, 1967.

Sacher, G.A., and Pearlman, N. Effects of total-body x-irradiation on rabbits. III. Effects on the leukocytes. In: Biological Effects of External X and Gamma Radiation. Ed. Raymond E. Zirkle, pp 290-316, McGraw-Hill, New York, 1954.

Saslaw, S. and Carlisle, H.N. Hematologic Response of monkeys to x-irradiation. Proc. Soc. Exp. Biol. Med. 105:60-62, 1960.

Siminovitch, L., Till, J.E., and McCulloch, E.A. Radiation responses of hemopoietic colony-forming cells derived from different sources. Radiation Res. 24:482-493, 1965.

Smith, W.W., Alderman, I.M., Schneider, C.A., and Cornfield, J. Effect of pretreatment with colchicine or a colchicine derivative on hemopoiesis in irradiated mice. Radiation Res. 19:621-627, 1963.

Stadler, J., and Gowen, J.W. Contributions to survival made by body cells of genetically differentiated strains of mice following x-irradiations. In: The Biological Bulletin, Vol. 112, Managing Ed. Donald P. Costello, Lancaster Press, Lancaster, Pa. 1957, pp. 400-421.

Stoner, R.D., and Bond, V.P. Antibody formation by transplanted bone marrow, spleen, lymph node and thymus cells in irradiated recipients. J. Immunol. 91:185-192, 1963.

Stoner, R.D., and Bond, V.P. Antibody formation by transplanted bone marrow, spleen, lymph nodes and thymus cells in irradiated recipients. J. Immun. 91(2):185-96, 1963.

Storer, J.B., Harris, P.S., Furchner, J.E., and Langham, W.H. The relative biological effectiveness of various ionizing radiations in mammalian systems. Radiation Res. 6:188-288, 1957.

Sugahara, T., Tanaka, T., Nagata, H., Man-I, M., and Kikuchi, K. Variation in radiosensitivity of mice in relation to their physiological conditions. Comparative Cellular and Species Radiosensitivity, Eds. V.P. Bond, and T. Sugahara, pp 30-41, Igaku Shoin Ltd., Tokyo, Japan, 1969.

Swift, M.N., Taketa, S.T., and Bond, V.P. Regionally fractionated x-irradiation equivalent in dose to total-body exposure. Radiation Res. 1:241-252, 1954.

Taketa, S.T., Carsten, A.L., Cohn, S.H., Atkins, H.L., and Bond, V.P. Active bone marrow distribution in the monkey. Life Sciences 169-174, 1970, Pergamon Press (Gr. Brit.).

Taketa, S.T., Carsten, A.L., Cohn, S.H., Atkins, H.L., and Bond, V.P. Active bone marrow distribution in the monkey. Life Sciences, 169-174. Pergamon Press (Gr. Brit.), 1970.

Till, J.E., and McCulloch, E.A. A direct measurement of the radiation sensitivity of normal bone marrow cells. Radiation Res. 14:213-222, 1961.

Tsuchiya, T., Hayakawa, J., Tamanoi, I, Muramatsu, S. and Dei, T. The difference in erythropoietic recovery after irradiation in two strains of mice. In: Comparative Cellular and Species Radiosensitivity, Eds. V.P. Bond and T. Sugahara, Igaku Shoin Ltd. Tokyo, Japan, 1969, pp. 53-62.

Tsuya, A. Bond, V.P., Fliedner, T.M., and Feinendegen, L.E. Cellularity and deoxyribonucleic acid synthesis in bone marrow after total- and partial-body irradiation. Radiation Res. 14:618-632, 1961.

Tullis, J.L., Chambers, F.W., Morgan, J.E., and Zeller, J.H. Mortality in swine and dose distribution on studies in phantoms exposed to super voltage x-radiations. Naval Medical Research Institute Report, Project NM 006 012.04.32, Aug. 29, 1950.

Tullis, J.L., Tessmer, C.F., Cronkite, E.P., and Chambers, F.W. Jr. The lethal dose of total body x-ray irradiation in swine. Radiology 52:396-400, 1949.

Tyazhelova, V.G., and Akoev, I.G. Equivalent conditions of irradiation of mammals. In: Radiobiology, ERDA-tr-99, Vol. 15, No. 3, pp 103-107, 1975.

Udupa, K.B., Shields, W. and Chute, R.N. Variations in $LD_{50/30}$ in a strain of rats over 20 years. Health Physics 26:319-322, 1974, Pergamon Press, Printed in Northern Ireland.

Ueno, Y. Cellular kinetics in the mouse hemopoietic system after exposure to ionizing radiation. In: Comparative Cellular and Species Radiosensitivity. Eds. V.P. Bond, and T. Sugahara, pp. 102-111, Igaku Shoin Ltd., Tokyo, Japan, 1969.

Upton, A.C. The pathogenesis of the hemorrhagic state in radiation sickness: A review. Blood 11:1156-1163, 1955.

van Bekkum, D.W. Bone marrow transplantation and partial body shielding for estimating cell survival and repopulation. In: Comparative Cellular and Species Radiosensitivity. Eds. V.P. Bond- and T. Sugahara, pp 175-201, Igaku Shoin Ltd., Tokyo, Japan, 1969.

Wakisaka, G., Yamagishi, M., Hama, M., Adachi, K. and Tzawa, H. Hematopoietic death and its prevention by bone marrow transplantation in irradiated mice. In: Comparative Cellular and Species Radiosensitivity, Eds. V.P. Bond and T. Sugahara, pp 193-201, Igaku Shoin Ltd., Tokyo, Japan, 1969.

Yuhas, J.M. and Storer, J.P. The effect of age on two modes of radiation death and on hematopoietic cell survival in the mouse. Radiation Res. 32:596-605, 1967.

Yuhas, J.M., and Storer, J.B. On mouse strain differences in radiation resistance: Hematopoietic death and the endogenous colony-forming unit. Radiation Res. 39:608-622, 1969.

EARLY RADIATION MORTALITY AND RECOVERY
IN LARGE ANIMALS AND PRIMATES

E. J. Ainsworth[1], G. F. Leong[2], and E. L. Alpen[3]

Biology and Medicine Division
Lawrence Berkeley Laboratory
Berkeley, CA 94720

INTRODUCTION

The rationale for large animal studies on early radiation mortality concerns their greater similarity to man in terms of size, metabolic rate, differential counts in peripheral blood, and other physiological factors than is the case for rodents. The phylogenetic relationship between the Rhesus monkey and man provided the incentive to study that species. Because most studies had their origins from consideration of nuclear weapons effects, animal size and depth-dose considerations were important for both neutrons and photons. The rationale for and interest in large animal radiobiology prevailed from the late 1940's to the late 1960's, and much useful information was obtained. Thereafter, interest waned because of high procurement and maintenance costs, and the generally high hassle factor associated with large animal radiobiology. While important experiments with large animals were performed in many laboratories, the major centers were the UT-AEC Agricultural Research Laboratory (UT Farm), the U.S. Naval Radiological Defense Laboratory (NRDL), the Air Force Weapons Laboratory (AFWL), the School of Aviation Medicine (SAM), and the Los Alamos Scientific Laboratory (LASL), and the Armed Forces Radiobiological Research Institute (AFRRI). After the demise of NRDL, a project on sheep was transfered to the Stanford Research Institute (SRI), and very important work proceeded there until about 1974. For reasons that will be obvious later, it is fair to say that more is known about the radiation responses of sheep to photons and neutrons, under a variety of exposure conditions, than any species other than rodents.

In the time and space assigned, we will provide only a brief overview of large animal responses, identify where relevant data reside, and present some results not readily available in the open scientific literature. Emphasis is placed on presenting data collected during the final years of NRDL's existence that were not included in reviews by Ainsworth et al. (1) and Page (2) in 1968. We also

---

[1] Formerly Head, Mammalian Radiobiology Section, U.S. Naval Radiobiological Defense Laboratory (NRDL).

[2] Formerly, Chief, Cellular Radiobiology Branch, USNRDL. Present address: 146 Atherton Ave., Atherton, CA 94025

[3] Formerly, Head, Biology and Medicine Division, USNRDL.

88

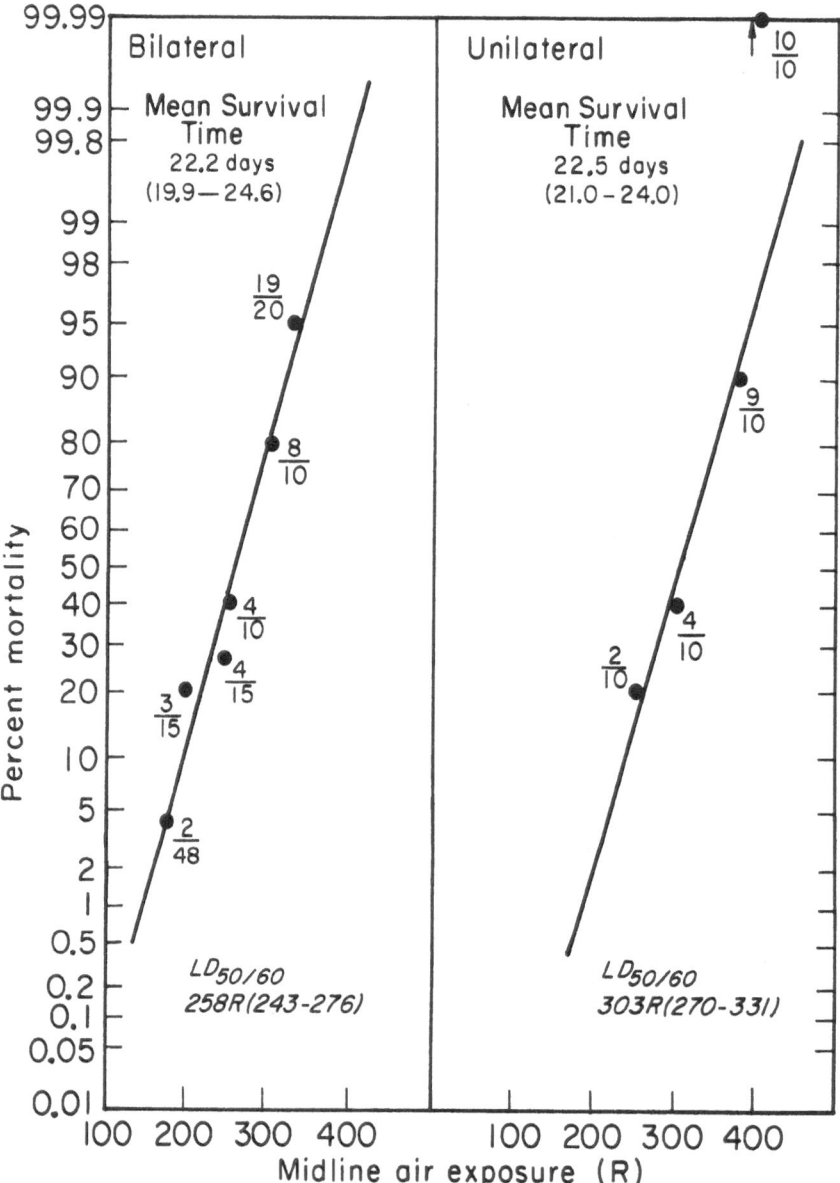

Figure 1 - Dose-response curves for Bilateral and Unilateral X-Irradiation of Sheep (1 MVP). The fraction by each point represents the number dying over the number exposed. The 95% confidence intervals are shown in parentheses. From Taylor et al. (11).

consider in detail data collected by Krebs and Jones on sheep at SRI (3), and recovery results on Rhesus monkeys collected by Eltringham at SAM (4) that will be published in the open literature.

The problems unique to large animal radiobiology and interpretation of the results were commented on specifically by Page (2). Beyond special facility requirements for holding and irradiation, several other matters are important. They include high genetic heterogeneity, variations in size, procurement of animals from different sources, health status in terms of microbial or parasitic pedigrees, variations in age, and maintenance of animals under circumstances where they are exposed to ambient weather conditions; all these contribute to variability. Additionally, variations in photon and neutron dosimetry, and estimation of dose at the midline or at some other location provides a challenge for comparing results from different laboratories. Sample sizes were often small, experiments were often unreplicated, and dose-response curves were often shallow, especially in split-dose studies.

Early Radiation Lethality

The term early radiation lethality is used here to denote the "hematopoietic syndrome" where animals succumb characteristically between 2 and 8 weeks following completion of radiation exposure. Some contribution from intestinal damage cannot be precluded, especially in animals exposed to neutrons, but the cause of death is largely attributed to hematopoietic failure. Burros and rabbits have some unique problems with a cardiovascular shock syndrome within minutes or hours after irradiation.

Following careful consideration of their adequacy as regards uniformity of exposure and dosimetry, Page summarized the data available in 1968 (2). They are too extensive to be considered here and many are available in the literature. Other subsequent relevant publications concern early mortality of miniature pigs to mixed neutron-gamma radiation (5). Broerse et al. have described the neutron LD_{50} for Rhesus monkeys (6), and Norris et al. reported the gamma ray $LD50/30$ for beagles (7). The response of 3-year-old adult female Columbia-Rambouillet sheep to pulsed mixed neutron-gamma radiation from a Godiva-type reactor was documented by T. S. Mobley et al (8). Mobley et al. also reported on 3-5 day lethality in sheep exposed unilaterally to ^{60}Co gamma rays and his report refers to earlier studies conducted at AFWL to define, comparatively, the role of intestinal and marrow damage in sheep exposed to pulsed neutron/gamma radiation or ^{60}Co gamma radiation (9,10).

Because prompt radiation from a nuclear weapon provides for unilateral exposure, considerable interest existed on how LD_{50} is influenced in various species when exposure is unilateral rather than omni-directional. Page summarized the data available in 1968 for sheep and dogs (2) and cited work in progress on gamma-irradiated sheep by Taylor. The dose-response curves from Taylor et al. for unilaterally and bilaterally irradiated sheep are shown in Figure 1 (11).

Table 1 - Dose Response and Mortality Data for Swine Following ^{60}Co Gamma Irradiation. From Taylor et al. (13)

Exposure Rate (R/hr)	Midline air Exposure (R)	Mortality No. Dead/No. Exposed	Days of Death
651	281	2/12	19,20
	351	5/12	17,18,19,29,30
	375	2/12	15,19
	375	9/12	12x2,13,14x2, 15x2,16,21
	469	9/12	13,16x3,17x3, 20,22
	565	11/12	11x2,12,13x3, 14x2,15x2,18
275	450	0/11	-
	475	0/12	-
	524	10/12	15,16,17x4, 18x2,19,24
	839	12/12	14x4,16,17x2 18x3, 19x2
30	600	1/10	15
	750	5/11	14,15x2,18,24
	900	3/10	11,12,14
	1000	8/12	10x2, 11x2, 13x2, 14x2
	1100	11/11	9,10x3,11x2, 12x4,15
	1350	4/4	9x3,15
4	930	1/12	14
	1000	1/12	10
	1200	3/12	12,13x2
	1550	1/10	18
	1800	0/9	-
	2015	5/10[a]	7x2,8x2,14
	2350	4/9[b]	2,4,29
	2800	2/7[c]	2,15

[a] 24 animals were put in the exposure field at the beginning of the exposure. Three died prior to exposure to 2015 R. Ten animals removed for 30 day observation after 2015 R. See Footnote c.

[b] 12 animals were put in the exposure field at the beginning of the exposure. Three died prior to exposure to 2350 R. The remaining nine animals removed for 30 day observation after 2350 R.

[c] Of the 11 animals remaining in the exposure field after 2015 R, four died prior to exposure to 2800 R. The remaining seven animals were removed for 30 day observation after 2800 R.

While the sample sizes and number of doses producing less than 100% mortality are meager, and the LD_{50}'s are not significantly different, the LD_{50} increase was of the order of 20%. In an attempt to elucidate differences in $LD_{50/60}$ values determined for Columbia-Rambouillet sheep at NRDL and AFWL, respectively, (9,10) Taylor et al. defined the relationship between body width and body weight for the sheep used at NRDL (11). Taylor et al. used a hematopoietic stem cell model proposed by Bond and Robinson to predict LD_{50} differences between bilaterally and unilaterally exposed sheep as a function of animal size (12). Using data on sheep, swine, and dog bilaterally or unilaterally exposed, they considered fractional stem cell survival at measured LD_{50} values, and alternatively, estimated how stem cell D_0 must vary among the 3 species to provide for equal stem cell survival at the measured LD_{50}s.

Early Radiation Lethality: Low and High Dose Rate Effects

Dose rate connotes relationship between physical dose and time. Often, dose rate refers to the instantaneous rate where no intervals of radiation-free time are involved. As used here, dose rate refers to instantaneous rate; clearly, low dose rates are accompanied by an increase in overall exposure time to deliver the dose and produce injury sufficient to produce early radiation mortality associated with hematopoietic failure. The data available in 1968 on several large animal species and primates were also summarized by Page (2).

The NRDL experience on dose rate effects in swine was summarized by Ainsworth (1). Included were unpublished results from Taylor et al.   Tables 1 and 2 present the mortality, survival time, and LD_{50} estimates from Taylor et al. (13). Results at 275 R/hr. were insufficient for precise estimation of LD_{50}; at 4 R/hr. the mortality response was not strikingly dose-dependent and a few animals died during the course of irradiation before programmed exposures were completed. The observation that animals died during protracted exposures is not surprising because the opportunity to express population variations in recovery potential is maximized when exposures are protracted over long periods of time. The single dose LD_{50} for ^{60}Co gamma radiation, 381 R, compares favorably with a value of 399 R for 1 MvP x-ray reported by Nachtwey et al. (14). The relative effect of dose rate on early radiation mortality in sheep and swine is shown by the following comparison: reducing the dose rate from about 655 to 3.6 R/hr. increased the LD_{50} in sheep from 237 to 495 R, a factor of about 2.0 while in swine the LD_{50} increased to about 3400 R, a factor approaching 9.0. Even using the lower 95% confidence limit for the LD_{50} at 4 R/hr. in swine yields an estimated LD_{50} increase of a factor approaching 6.0. Brown and Cragle also commented on the rapid recovery from radiation damage in swine in comparison with other species with which they have had experience at the UT Farm, so data available in the literature provide a consistant appraisal of the high recovery capacity of swine (15).

The pulsed radiation characteristics and high dose rates associated with prompt radiation from nuclear weapons stimulated

Table 2 - Influence of Exposure Rate on the LD_{50} of Swine after ^{60}Co Gamma Irradiation. From Taylor et al. (13).

Exposure Rate R/Hr	$LD_{50/30}$	Slope[a]	x^{2}[b]	30 Day Mean Survival Time (Days)	
651	381 R (341-423)[c]	3.406	8.271	16.34	(14.96-17.73)[c]
275	500 R	-	-	17.09	(16.09-18.10)
30	849 R (752-936)	4.039	6.857	12.47	(11.36-13.58)
4	3444 R (2259-6107)[d]	1.014	5.665	11.00	(7.42-14.58)

[a]Slope of exposure response curve in terms of probit of mortality per log_{10} of the exposure in (R).

[b]Linearity chi square value.

[c]95% confidence interval.

[d]Using the data from Table 1 for the animals surviving the predetermined exposure.

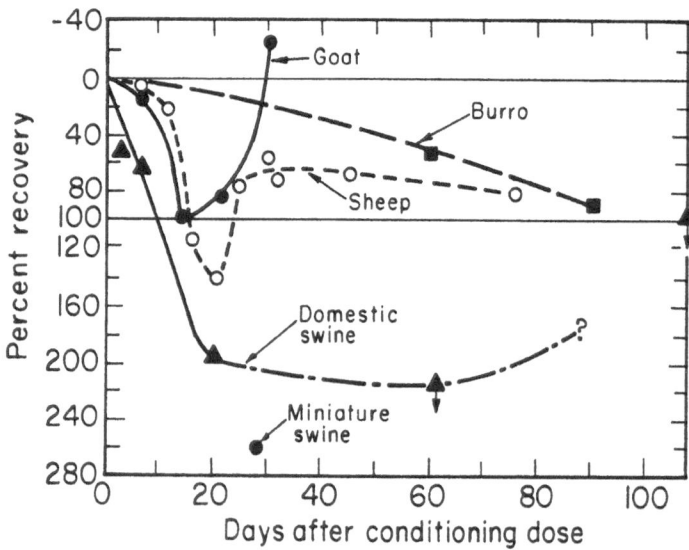

Figure 2 - Interspecies comparison of recovery patterns after sublethal conditioning doses (2/3 $LD_{50/30-60}$) as evaluated by the split-dose technique. From Taylor et al. (20).

research on high dose rates in the range of 10^6 - 10^8 rad/min.
Reports by Ainsworth et al. with dogs and Hauver et al. with sheep
indicated no differences in LD_{50} between pulsed radiation and radiation delivered at 10-40 rad/min [16,17]. Other information on sheep
exposed to pulsed fission spectrum radiations is available in a report
by Mobley et al. [18].

Recovery from Radiation Injury Evaluated by Split-Dose Lethality

Page reviewed the status of split-dose lethality studies in large
animals and primates where it was inferred that hematopoietic failure
was the principal cause of death [2]. The goat data were published
subsequently by Taylor et al. [19]. Regarding the primate response,
we are indebted to Dr. James Eltringham for providing the Rhesus
monkey data from a manuscript in preparation for presentation here.
He presented the results available in 1967 at the Radiation Research
Society Meeting in Puerto Rico [4]. The Macaca mulatta obtained from
commercial suppliers ranged in weight from 1.8-4.3 kg and were housed
individually. They were irradiated with 60 cobalt gamma radiation at
54.6 rad/min. (on the axis of rotation) and rotated at 3 rpm in a
perforated 15 cm plexiglass cylinder with 6 mm thick walls. No
anesthesia was used. Monkeys used in the single and split-dose studies were irradiated in the knee chest position. The conditioning dose
(D_c) was 400 midline tissue rad. The single and split dose results
are shown in Table 3.

In brief, the major features of the interspecies recovery comparison described by Page are that the pig and dog recover relatively
rapidly, the few data points with the burro are consistent with relatively slow recovery, and the monkey shows only a transient recovery
within 6 weeks [2]. Goats and particularly sheep recover more slowly
than dogs and pigs, and sheep may experience a multi-day delay in
initiating recovery. Page described three phases of the sheep recovery curve namely, an initial lag, a rapid recovery phase with an
overshoot to acquired radioresistance, and subsequent reexpression of
residual injury [2]. The original data must be consulted for critical
assessment of the statistical significance of changes in radiosensitivity. Regarding acquired radiosensitivity, the $LD_{50/60}$ for sheep
challenged at 20 days after a D_c of 165 R differed significantly from
the LD_{50} for animals challenged at 24, 30, 31, or 45 days after irradiation. The split-dose $LD_{50/60}$ at 20 days 324 R (271-399) was also
significantly higher than the single dose LD_{50} of 237 R (215-257).
The most impressive acquired radioresistance was in swine where the
LD_{50} for unconditioned controls was 399 R (371-424) and the LD_{50} rede-
termined at 20 days after a D_c of 265 R was 654 (594-758) [14].
Limited additional data collected at 61 and 107 days were consistent
with a sustained acquired radioresistance [14]. Taylor et al. inde-
pendently confirmed the acquired radioresistance by demonstrating that
miniature swine exposed to ^{60}Co gamma radiation at AFRRI had an LD_{50}
of 477 rad at 28 days after a D_c of 150 rad; where the single dose
$LD_{50/30}$ was 237 rad [20]. The single recovery point determined for
miniature swine is compared with domestic swine, sheep, burros, and
goats in Fig. 2. This figure also shows goat data collected by Taylor

Table 3 - Single and Split-Dose LD_{50} Estimates For <u>Macaca Mulatta</u>
Exposed to ^{60}Co Gamma Radiation. From Eltringham (4)
and personal communication, 1983.

Re-Exposure Time (Days)	$LD_{50/30}$* (Rads)	LD50/60 (Rads)	No.	Percent Residual Injury(%)
0	644 (613-678)	644 (613-678)	90	--
7	317 (259-369)	293 (234-351)	94	87 (71-102)
14	386 (280-444)	381 (292-432)	86	66 (50-83)
21	249 (186-292)	205 (98-258)	90	110 (92-128)
28	183 (168-197)	169 (147-188)	96	119 (110-128)
42	253 (164-312)	213 (85-279)	73	108 (87-129)

*Values in ( ) = 95% C. L.
D_1 - 400 Rad

TABLE 4 - MORTALITY OF SHEEP CONDITIONED WITH 155 R ^{60}CO AT 8.5 R PER MINUTE AND IMMEDIATELY CHALLENGED WITH COBALT AT 3.85 R PER HOUR. FROM STILL ET AL. (21).

CHALLENGE EXPOSURE (R)	DEAD/TOTAL 30 DAYS	DEAD/TOTAL 60 DAYS	DAY OF DEATH	MST DAYS
65	1/10	1/10	25	25
150	0/10	0/10	----	> 60
185	8/10	9/10	12,18,20 X 5,24,32	20.7 (16.6 - 24.7)[a]
240	5/10	7/10	13,15 x 2, 19 x 2,32,35	21.1 (13.0 - 29.3)
270	10/13	10/13	17 x 2,18,19,20,21,22,23,25,27	20.9 (18.5 - 23.3)
350	13/14	14/14	15 x 3, 17 x 2, 18 x 3, 21 x 2, 23, 30 x 2,37	21.1 (17.2 - 24.9)
450	12/14	12/14	14 x 3, 15 x 3, 16,17, 18 x 3, 20	16.2 (14.9 - 17.4)
500	12/13	12/13	10, 13 x 3, 14 x 3,16,19,20, 21,23	15.8 (13.3 - 18.4)

Computed LD 50/60: 171 R (124 - 209)[a]

LD 10/60: 77 R (35 - 110)

LD 90/60: 379 R (303 - 569)

Slope: 1.605[b]

Coefficient of Variation: 0.689

Chi^2: 16.39

Mean Survival Time, all animals: 19.18 days (17.8 - 20.6)[a]

a - 95% confidence interval.
b - In terms of normal equivalent deviates (probit minus five) of percent mortality per unit natural logarithm of exposure.

TABLE 5 - MORTALITY OF SHEEP EXPOSED TO 1 MVP X-RAYS AT A RATE OF 7.5 R PER MINUTE. FROM STILL ET AL. (21).

CHALLENGE EXPOSURE (R)	DEAD/TOTAL 30 DAYS	DEAD/TOTAL 60 DAYS	DAY OF DEATH	MST DAYS
225[a]	0/10	0/10	----	> 60
240[b]	2/11	3/11	22,23,36	27 (7.6 - 46)[c]
275[a]	1/10	1/10	30	30
290[b]	4/11	4/11	21,23 x 2,25	23 (20.4 - 25.6)
325[a]	5/10	5/10	17,19,21,22,24	20.6 (17.3 - 23.9)
340[b]	8/11	9/11	19,21,22,23,24,25 x 2,26,38	24.8 (20.6 - 28.9)
375[a]	8/11	8/11	19 x 3,20,22,23 x 2,24	21.1 (19.4 - 22.9)

Computed LD50/60: 314 R (292 - 344)[c]

LD10/60: 238 R (189 - 262)

LD90/60: 414 R (369 - 552)

Slope: 4.60[d]

Coefficient of Variation: 0.219

Chi^2: 7.034

Mean Survival Time, all animals: 23.3 days (21.6 - 25.0)[c]

a - Indicates animals selected from one purchase lot.
b - Indicates animals selected from a different purchase lot.
c - 95% confidence interval.
d - In terms of normal equivalent deviates (probit minus five) of percent mortality per unit natural logarithm of exposure.

et al. subsequent to the Page presentation in 1968. Note that both the goat and Rhesus return to a radiosensitive state, consistent with no recovery, following at least one earlier determination that is consistent with appreciable recovery.

Recovery: Acute Injury Followed by Low Level Exposures

The split dose recovery curve in sheep, indicating a significant time lag in the initiation of recovery after a conditioning dose (D_c) given at a high dose rate (HDR) provided the rationale to pursue studies on the effect of low level irradiation immediately following a HDR D_c. The hypothesis was the injury produced by the D_c would impair recovery from radiation injury produced at low dose rates. Still et al. showed that when sheep were given a D_c of 155 R (510 R/hr.) and placed in a chronic radiation field at 3.85 R/hr., the $LD_{50/60}$ was 171 R (Table 4). Groups of animals were then exposed at 3.85 R/hr. until preselected doses were given and they were removed from the radiation field. The highest (chronic) challenge dose used, 500 R was given within the 7-day "lag period." Because the single dose LD_{50} for animals given single doses at the rate of 450 R/hr. was 314 R (Table 5), and the LD_{50} for animals that received the high dose rate D_c followed by chronic exposure was 326 R, the inference was that recovery during low-level exposure was largely inhibited (21).

Krebs and Jones followed up on this observation when NRDL closed and the sheep program was moved to SRI (3). Their experiments were designed to determine what dose, given at HDR, was necessary to inhibit recovery processes in animals exposed to a dose of 134 R at 3.8 R/hr. Rather than give graded doses at 3.8 R/hr., with an attendant variable increase in exposure time as did Still et al. (21), Jones and Krebs challenged animals with graded doses given at HDR after the chronic exposure of 134 R was received. The LD_{50}'s, expressed as total doses (HDR D_c, plus 134 R chronically received, plus the challenged LD_{50}) are shown in Table 6, Series 2. The appropriate single dose LD_{50} comparison is shown in Table 6, Series 1. The LD_{50} was not as high as expected in "control" animals that received the D_c of zero R, and while the total dose LD_{50}s were lower in animals that received the HDR D_c's, none of the differences was significant. The point made by Krebs and Jones was when chronic exposures immediately follow a single exposure at HDR, it would seem prudent to consider that the chronic exposure was also received at a HDR (3). Because none of the LD_{50}'s in Table 6, Series 2 differed from the single dose LD_{50}, this interpretation seems appropriate. A complicating factor in the Still et al. experiment was that because of the graded nature of the chronically administered challenged doses, the time available for animals to recover during the chronic exposure ranged from less than 1 day to approximately 5.5 days (21). The acute-chronic-acute experiment designed by Krebs and Jones eliminated that variable. It is likely that the inherent variability of the sheep model system was such that the appreciable difference in recovery during chronic exposure at 3.8 R/hr. could not be detected where the total chronic exposure was only 134 R given over 36 hrs.

Table 6: Early Radiation Mortality in Sheep Exposed to ^{60}Co Gamma Radiation. From Krebs and Jones (3).

Series	Experiment	Conditions	Other Comments	No. Exper.	Doses	N	LD50/60(R)	MST
1)	Single Dose LD50/60	DR 561-578 R/hr	D_1 0 R	3	6	180	273 (257-289)	25.4 ±.6
2)	Inhibition of Recover by acute exposure (Acute-Chronic-Acute Experimental Design)	D_1 at 561-578 R/hr (0, 9.1, 45 R)	D_1 0 R	1	5	60	298 (254-285)	25.1 +4.3
		D_2 at 3.8 R/hr (134 R) Challenge at 561-578 R/hr	D_1 9.1 R	1	5	60	278 (259-297)	24.3 ±2.8
			D_1 45 R	1	5	60	270 (281-316)	22.3 +2.5
3)	Injury Accumulation at 0.45 R/hr and LD50/60 prediction	ADR 9.83 R/22.5 hr/d 74 days = 727 R challenge at 514 R/hr	Estimated LD50/60 at 514 R/hr 273 R Estimated LD50/60 at 0.45 R/hr 1713 R	1	5	58	157 (118-196)	28.5 +3.1

Table 6: Continued

Series	Experiment	Conditions	Other Comments	No. Exper.	Doses	N	LD50/60(R)	MST
4)	LD50/60 at 0.9 or 3.6 R/hr	ADR ~ 20 R/d Chronic/Fractionated	0.9 Rx22.5 hrs	1	5	60	1252 (1149-1354)	19.1 + 4.8
		Terminated Exposure	3.6 R x 5.3 hrs	1	3	36	1251 (863-1639)	---
5)	LD50/60 Chronic-Chronic 152 hrs/wk	ADR ~30 R/d (27 or 34) 140 R at 3.4 R/hr (41 hrs)	100 R at 0.9/hr (111 hrs)	1	4	60	680 (543-817)	16.4 +4.9
	Weekly doses of 190 or 240 R	140 R 3.4 R (41 hrs)	50 R at 0.45 R/hr (111 hrs)	1	4	60	920 (823-1018)	14.8 +5.4
6)	LD50/60 Chronic at 140 R/wk	ADR ~ 23 R/d 3.4 R/hr (41 hrs/wk)	Exposed 2 d/wk	2	4	71	936 (836-1036)	16.7 +6.0
7)	LD50/60 Chronic 240 R/2 wks	ADR ~ 24 R/d 3.4R/hr (82 hrs/2wks) plus 140 to some groups	Exposed 3-5 d/ 2wks	1	6	70	1131 (1007-1220)	2.8 +7.5

Table 6: Continued

Series	Experiment	Conditions	Other Comments	No. Exper.	Doses	N	LD50/60(R)	MST
8)	LD$_{50/60}$ Chronic 153 R/2wks	ADR ~ 13 R/d 10.3 R/hr(15 hrs/2wks) 2wks	Exposed <1 d/	2	3/4	103	745 (640-850)	27.1 ±7.5
9)	LD$_{50/60}$ Fractionated Doses - 5 wks	34, 44, or 54 R at 607 R/hr 3 times/wk	Expected Single Dose LD$_{50}$ 261 R	1	3	36	522 (438-607)	16.8 ±6.6
10)	Residual Injury at 90 or 180 d	Survivors of exposures at 0.45-3.4 R/hr; reirradiated at 465-565 R/hr	Challenge at 90 d	4	3/4	155	140-180 R[a]	27-35
	High dose rate challenge		Challenge at 180 d	1	3	35	171[a] (142-199)	37.2 ±6.6
11)	Residual Injury at 90 d Low dose rate challenge	Survivors of Exposures at 0.45-3.4 R/hr; reirradiated with 121 R/wk at 10.5 R/hr (11.5 hrs)	Begin challenge at 90 d	1	4	36	553[b] (491-616)	19.8 ±6.2

a With no residual injury, expected (dose rate adjusted) LD$_{50/60}$ range is 268-281 R.
b With no residual injury, LD50/60, is estimated at 659 R; direct measurement.

Other results reported by Krebs and Jones bear directly on the question of recovery after doses given at HDR, and possibly, the effects of dose/fraction on recovery potential. When exposures of 34, 44, or 54 R were given 3 times/wk. at 607 R/hr. and the exposures terminated after 5 weeks, the LD_{50} was estimated at 522 R, a value approximately twice the single dose LD_{50} (Table 6, Series 9). While the series involved only a small number of animals and was not replicated, the results are consistent with the interpretation that at "low" doses per fraction given at HDR, recovery proceeds. They pointed out that the increment in $LD_{50/60}$, approximately a factor of 2.0, is similar to that observed for mice when HDR fractions were administered over 4 weeks (3). As will be discussed further below, "low doses" given at high or low rates may actuate recovery systems.

Recovery During and Following Exposure at Low Dose Rates:

Low dose rate is used here to denote exposures given at 12 R/hr. or below in either a continuous mode or under circumstances where the chronic exposures are interrupted and the animals are provided radiation-free time. The NRDL program considered various exposure scenarios relevant to military applications, one of which was exposure in a fallout field under hypothetical circumstances where the exposure (rate) was constant. Experimental questions, some of which have been considered above, concern lethal effects at low dose rates (LDR), the rates of injury accumulation or recovery during exposure, and the pattern of recovery upon exit from a fallout field. Limited data were accumulated with swine, a pilot experiment was conducted with the Rhesus, and an extensive data set exist for sheep.

Ainsworth et al. reviewed the NRDL swine and sheep data available in 1968 (1). The sheep data were published in the open literature (22-24). Also cited was work in progress by Taylor et al. concerning injury accumulation in swine exposed at LDR. The Taylor et al. data on $LD_{50/30}$ at low dose rates were considered previously in Tables 1 and 2, and the full extent of the data available on injury accumulation in swine exposed at 4 R/hr. are shown in Table 7 (13). Swine received a D_c of 250, 500, or 750 R and were challenged with the doses specified at about 600 R/hr. Sample sizes were small, the experiment was unreplicated, and the LD_{50} following a D_c of 750 R could only be estimated. Clearly, caution is prudent in terms of conclusions regarding injury accumulation rate(s), or conversely, recovery rates during chronic exposure. Injury accumulation did not appear to increase with the size of the conditioning exposure. Interpreted cautiously, and only qualitatively, results indicate a lower injury accumulation or greater recovery potential in swine than in sheep. This is consistent with early observations by Brown and Cragle (15). Interpreted liberally, the results could indicate a non-linear rate of injury accumulation such that injury accumulates more rapidly during the first 2.5 days of exposure (250 R) than during the subsequent 5 days of exposure necessary to achieve the total D_c of 750 R. While the concept that time, injury, and injury rate may influence actuation of recovery systems, the NRDL data on swine are insufficient to firmly support a conclusion other than the recovery rate in swine,

Table 7 - Injury Accumulation in Swine Following ^{60}Co Gamma Irradiation-Dose Response and Mortality Data. Adapted from Taylor et al. (13).

Conditioning Exposure at 4 R/hr[a]	Challenge Exposure (R)[b]	Mortality No. Dead/No. Exposed	LD50/30(R)	Roentgen Equivalent Injury (R)[e]	Days of Death	Mean Survival Time
250	140	0/12	-			
	210	2/12	247		24,26	
	257	7/12	(224-286)	134	13,18x2,19x3,28	18.3 (16.3-20.2)
	376	11/11			12,13,15x2,16x2, 17x2,19x2,22	
500	142	0/12			-	
	211	3/9	228	153	15x2, 17	17.1 (14.4-19.7)
	284	10/11	(194-258)		12,13,15x2,16x2, 18,19,22,29	
750	96	1/11	206	175	14	13.1 (11.1-15.2)
	239	7/11			8,12,13x2,14, 15,16	

a - Midline air exposure.

b - Challenge exposures delivered at 600 R/hr.

c - Values in parentheses are 95% confidence limits.

d - Pooled value for all decedents at each challenge time

e - LD50/30 at 650 R/hr. - LD50/30 determined following the conditioning exposure.

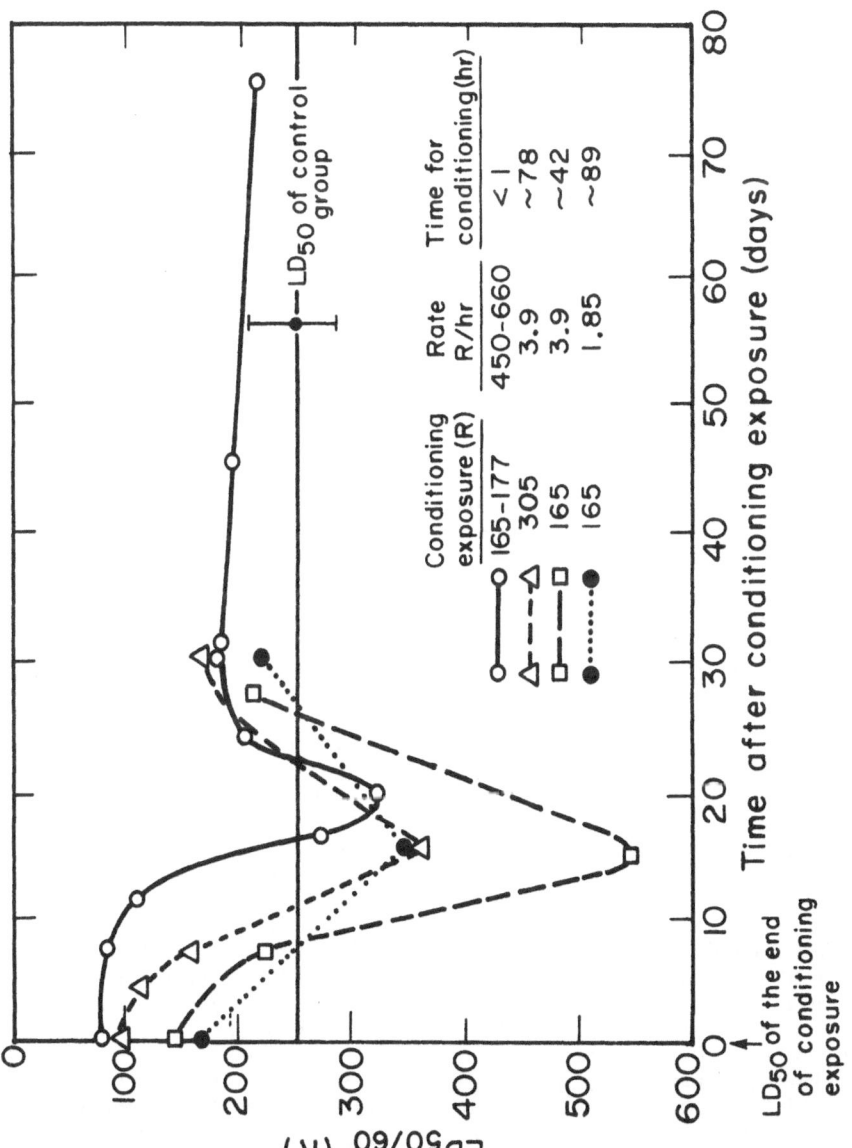

Figure 3 - Split-dose LD$_{50}$'s for sheep at various times after completion of either an acute or protracted conditioning exposure. From Page et al. (24).

2.4-3.7 R/hr., is probably greater than the recovery rate in sheep, 1.7-2 R/hr., at exposures of 4.0 or 3.6 R/hr., respectively.

The initial injury accumulation studies in sheep were reported by Hanks et al. (22). Sheep were given an exposure of 165 R at rates of 0.5, 0.95, 1.85, or 3.9 R/hr. and were challenged essentially immediately at HDR. The results showed no injury accumulation and a trend toward slight resistance at dose rates of 0.5 or 0.95 R/hr. Significant injury accumulation and significantly reduced $LD_{50/60}$s were found when 165 R was administered at 1.85 or 3.9 R/hr. Recovery from injury accumulated during chronic exposures to 165 R at 1.9 or 3.9 R/hr. were described by Page et al. and Ainsworth et al. (2,1), and the results are shown in Figure 3. Recovery, as indicated by returning to a normal $LD_{50/60}$ appeared to proceed rapidly, possibly without as much of a lag that occurs after a D_c given at a HDR. The acquired radioresistance observed at 15 days after completion of the exposure at 3.9 R/hr. was the greatest observed in sheep and occurred earlier than when the D_c was given at a HDR. Figure 3 also shows the return toward a normal LD_{50} following chronic exposure to 305 R at 3.9 R/hr. where the injury accumulated was similar to that expected from a single dose of 165 R given at an HDR. The results indicated the lag is probably less and the acquired radioresistance occurs earlier when the D_c was given at a LDR. In all groups the trend was toward reexpression of residual injury at the few intervals studied after 20 days. In sum, the results indicate that recovery systems are actuated under conditions of chronic exposure at LDR's and the return toward a normal $LD_{50/60}$ may occur more rapidly when the D_c is given at a LDR. Differences in mean survival time, some statistically significant, among groups given D_c's at different dose rates and challenged at different times were reported by Page et al. (23). The trend among challenged animals was that survival times were shorter at 20 days or before than thereafter.

Data on injury accumulation in sheep are more generous than with swine, but precise estimation of rates is more than the data can realistically provide. The injury accumulation data in sheep are documented fully (1,22-24) so suffice it to make only a few points based on the summary shown in Fig. 4. The figure indicates estimated amounts of injury accumulation from studies where animals were challenged after receiving D_c's at dose rates of 1.9 or 3.6 R/hr. and were challenged at HDR's. Also, it is assumed that the injury at the LD_{50} levels measured directly at LDR is equivalent to 237 R, namely the LD_{50} determined at a HDR. There are only three points on the curve at an exposure rate of 1.9 R/hr. Fig. 4 shows alternate ways of fitting the data where neither fit can be excluded on rigorous statistical grounds because of the meager results. Speculation by Ainsworth et al. was that the injury accumulation rate, or conversely the recovery rate, could be influenced by the exposure rate such that the recovery rate was higher at the higher exposure rate (1). Subsequent data and their interpretation by Krebs and Jones supports this concept (3).

The results in Fig. 4 on injury accumulation in sheep are clearly inadequate to define linearity or non-linearity of injury accumula-

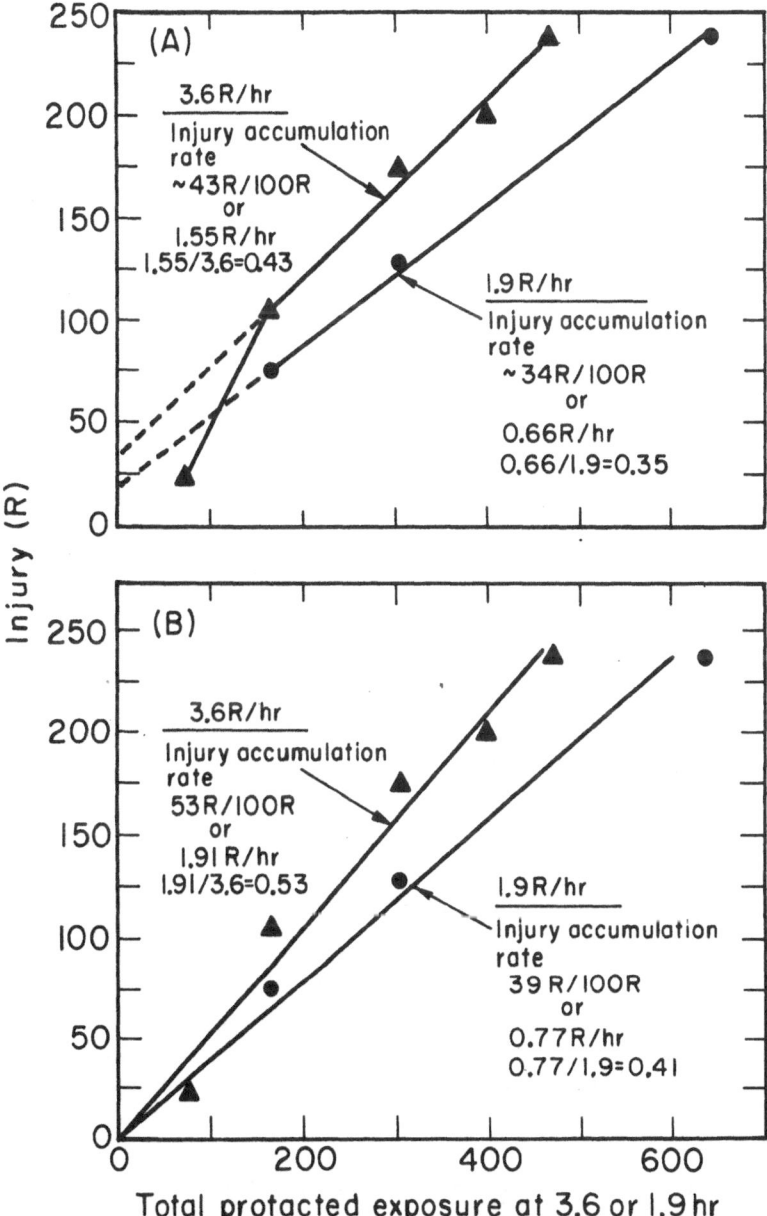

Figure 4 - Injury accumulation in sheep exposed at 3.6 or 1.9 R/hr. This figure illustrates two ways of fitting the data; in (A) the curves are not forced to a y intercept of 0, whereas, in (B) a y intercept of 0 is assumed. From Ainsworth et al. (1).

tion, especially at total exposures less than 165 R. Accepting injury estimates at face value, the results at D_c of 75 and 165 R received at 3.6 R/hr. could generously be interpreted as indicating considerable recovery when the exposure was 75 R and a lower recovery at an exposure of 165 R., i.e., an increasing rate of injury accumulation with dose and time to 165 R. This could also be generously interpreted as saturation of the recovery system as injury accrues. This interpretation is not totally inconsistent with other results at lower exposure rates. Hanks et al. reported no injury accumulation with total exposures of 165 R at 0.5 and 0.95 R/hr. (22), but unpublished data from Page et al. presented by Ainsworth et al. indicated significant injury accumulation at 0.9-1 R/hr. when animals were challenged at an HDR after protracted exposures totalling 642 or 702 R (1). Similarly, no injury was detected at 0.5 R/hr. when the total exposure was 165 R (22), but Krebs and Jones found significant injury accumulation after 74 days at 0.45 R/hr. when animals were challenged at a HDR (Table 6, Series 3). The paucity of data provide the opportunity for various interpretations of the injury accumulation results at exposure rates of 1.0 or 0.5 R/hr. including a non zero injury accumulation after a total of 165 R as reported by Hanks et al (22). Suffice it to say that the hypothesis concerning saturation of recovery systems when injury is accumulated at low exposures has not been adequately tested, but remains a very interesting possibility.

Information on injury accumulation in the Rhesus monkey at an exposure rates of 0.5 R/hr. is even more meager, but interesting and important results were collected by Eltringham, and he has kindly permitted their inclusion here. Monkeys received a total exposure of 435 R of ^{60}Co gamma radiation at about 15 R/23-hour-day (about 0.7 R/hr.) Twenty-eight days after completion of the chronic exposures, groups of 6 animals were challenged at about 55 R/hr. The 60-day mortality was 3/6 at 350 rad, 4/6 at 450 rad, 5/6 at 550 rad, and 6/6 at 650 rad. Conceding immediately their preliminary nature, the results suggest the presence of residual radiation injury. With the reported single dose LD_{50} of 644 rad, one might infer 200-300 R of remaining injury (Table 3). All that may be cautiously inferred is that injury was present, but its quantitative relationship to the injury accumulation during the chronic exposures, or to excursions in recovery and expression of injury following completion of the exposure, cannot be ascertained. However, it seems plausible that some level of injury accumulated in the Rhesus during chronic exposure.

Early Radiation Lethality in Sheep:
Effect of Instantaneous Rates and Radiation Free Time

Total dose, dose rate, duration of exposure, and radiation-free time provide the experimentalist with confounded variables providing for a lifes' work. Krebs and Jones dealt with this challenge directly in an excellent series of experiments and provided data, sometimes meager, to test hypothesis regarding prediction of early radiation lethality in sheep based on the concept of averaged daily rate (ADR). The comprehensive 1975 report by Krebs and Jones details their conceptual and mathematical approaches using "exposure dose rate" (EDR) and averaged dose rate (ADR) to analyze their sheep data and the data of others with mice, swine, and dogs (3). That document should be consulted by those seriously interested in interspecies comparisons and modeling of early radiation lethality.

In brief, EDR pertains to what has been referred to above as dose rate effects for production of early radiation lethality. The concept of ADR pertains to the integral of total exposure divided by the full interval over which the exposure was given, i.e., the beginning of the exposure to the end of the exposure, irrespective of radiation free time. Specific experiments were designed by Krebs and Jones to test the ADR concept and several series are summarized in Table 6. Implicit in the ADR concept is the hypothesis that early radiation mortality in sheep is predictable based on daily averaged ADR (in R/day), and this further embodies implicit assumptions about recovery rates at the dose rates used. Consideration here will be restricted to 2 experiments summarized in Table 6, one of which appears to support the ADR concept while the other does not. In Series 4 sheep received daily irradiation to preselected total levels of exposure and were removed from the radiation field. ADR's of about 20 R/day were achieved by exposing animals at 0.9 R/hr. for about 22.5 hours or at 3.6 R for about 5.3 hrs. Although the data at the higher dose rate are meager and there were too few decedents for computation of mean survival time, the LD_{50}'s of about 1250 R indicate instantaneous dose rate and radiation free time had no effect on early radiation mortality. Also, LD_{50}'s in the range of 930 and 1110 R were observed where ADR's were about 23 and 24 R/day and the radiation-free time was progressively greater. These results are shown in Table 6, Series 6 and 7). Series 5 presents results at an ADR of about 30 R/day (actually 27 or 34) where animals were exposed to weekly doses of 190 or 240 R in a total time of 152 hrs./week (16 hours of radiation-free time each week). The number of hours and exposures at 2 different rates are shown in Table 6. If it assumed that ADR's of 27 or 34 are really not different, and an averaged ADR of about 30 holds, the LD_{50}'s should have been similar, where in fact they differed significantly. The results are consistent with the interpretation that the rate of injury accumulation was lower for the group exposed to 0.5 R/hr. It should also be noted that the mean survival times tended to be shorter and the response more variable compared to decedents involved in the single dose studies at HDR. Further critical analysis of the ADR concept is beyond the scope of this presentation.

Residual Injury

In the context of split dose lethality studies, where the D_c is at high or low rates, residual injury connotes a greater than normal radiation sensitivity, i.e., a somewhat reduced LD_{50}. In rodents a value like 10% of the conditioning dose appears to apply. Because of the shallow nature of dose-response curves it is likely that many of the estimates of residual injury in rodents are derived from LD_{50} values that do not differ significantly from "normal." Krebs and Jones evaluated residual injury at 90 or 180 days in sheep that were survivors of exposures at 0.45 or 3.4 R/hr. The average dose to the various groups of animals was estimated, and the survivors were reirradiated with graded doses at HDR. Of considerable interest is their observation that the LD_{50} of challenged survivors was in the range of 140-180 R at both 90 and 100 days (meager data at 180 days), (see Table 6, Series 10). They estimated residual injury amounted to approximately 50% of the injury that remained at the conclusion of the chronic exposures. Residual injury was also estimated by subjecting survivors of exposures at LDR's to weekly doses of 121 R at 10.5 R/hr. (Table 6, Series 11) and they interpreted the data to indicate the chronic radiation challenge revealed approximately 20% of the injury remaining at the end of the initial chronic exposure persisted as residual injury. While the sample size in the group that was chronically challenged was small, Krebs and Jones indicated the estimate of residual injury was not independent of the experimental design used to estimate residual injury, namely HDR exposures or chronic exposures. They speculated the difference was related to actuation of the recovery system by the experimental design that involved chronic exposures; whereas, the same opportunity for actuation was not presented animals that were challenged at a HDR. In view of other results described above, their interpretation is quite plausible. Their results from the HDR challenge groups are quite adequate, their interpretation of results is cautious, and their results provide a significant invitation for further studies to define residual injury in sheep and other large animal species.

Conclusions

When large animals and primate studies of early radiation mortality were precipitiously terminated in the late 1960's or early 1970's species-dependent differences in sensitivity, effects of dose rate, and recovery processes had been defined. However, the cellular and physiological bases for observed differences were not revealed. Because the bone marrow syndrome is largely the issue, correlative interspecies research on bone marrow populations and cell kinetics should be informative. Relationships between radiation sensitivity and damage to various critical hematopoietic compartments remain to be determined under a variety of exposure conditions. Selective interspecies comparisons focusing on the hematopoietic system response to radiation will be informative and could be useful for predictive purposes if ethically and scientifically acceptable correlative information can be collected for man. Any experimental approach based on the concept that a single species will be revealed that is the singular surrogate for man will undoubtedly be credited with high marks for sheer folly. If new effort is to be directed to future interspecies comparison of early radiation mortality, an essential prerequisite is the critical evaluation, far more critical and estensive than provided here, of existing data and comprehensive consideration of results available on hematopoietic responses. A large body of data on lethality and hematopoietic responses in large animals exists. While many data are available in the open literature, some important results repose only in technical reports. Before proceeding with new research, critical assessments of all existing data should be conducted and the most critical scientific questions defined.

Acknowledgements

This contribution is dedicated to the late John S. Krebs, a long time travelling companion, office mate, colleague, and friend of E. J. Ainsworth and G. F. Leong. With pleasure we acknowledge the scientific ability, dedication, and hard work contributed by the following NRDL Investigators and members of the "NRDL Alumni Association," who served as Directors of the various projects that generated many of the data reported here: William Wisecup, Gerald Hanks, Norbert Page, James Taylor, Edwin Still, and D. Stuart Nachtwey. James Eltringham contributed materially by providing the Rhesus monkey data for inclusion in this document. David Jones kindly loaned his nearly last copy of the OCD report (3) to assist with our communication. The assistance of Victor Sevilla in typing the manuscript quickly is also gratefully acknowledged. This effort was supported by NASA Contract No. T3516G and DOE Contract No. DE-AC03-76SF00098.

References

1. Ainsworth, E. J., N. P. Page, J. F. Taylor, G. F. Leong, and E. T. Still, Dose-rate studies in sheep and swine. In: Symposium on Dose Rate Effects in Mammalian Radiation Biology, pp. 4.1-4.22. USAEC Report CONF 680410 (1968).

2. Page, N. P., The effect of dose protraction on radiation lethality of large animals. In: Symposium on Dose Rate Effects in Mammalian Radiation Biology, pp. 12.1-12.23. USAEC Report CONF 680410 (1968).

3. Krebs, J. S. and D. C. L. Jones. Radiobiology of large animals, Final Report for Contract DAHC20-70-C-0219 DCPA Work Unit 24310; SRI Project PYU-8150, June (1975).

4. Eltringham, J. R., Recovery of the Rhesus monkey from acute radiation exposure as evaluated by the split-dose technique: preliminary results. Rad. Res. 31: 533 (1967).

5. Wise, D. and C. L. Turbyfill, The acute mortality response of the miniature pig to pulsed mixed gamma-neutron radiations. Rad. Res. 41: 507-515 (1970).

6. Broerse, J. J. and D. W. van Bekkum, Mortality of monkeys after exposure to fission neutrons and the effect of autologous bone marrow transplantation. Int. J. Radiat. Biol., Vol. 34(3): 253-264 (1978).

7. Norris, W. P., T. E. Fritz, C. E. Rehfeld, and C. M. Poole, The response of the beagle dog to Cobalt-60 gamma radiation: Determination of the $LD_{50(30)}$ and description of associated changes. Rad. Res. 35: 681-708 (1968).

8. Mobley, T. S., R. L. Persing, and J. L. Terry, Effects of various dose rates of mixed neutron-gamma radiations on the $LD_{50(60)}$ response of sheep. U. S. Air Force Weapons Laboratory, USAFWL-TR-71-5, September (1974).

9. Mobley, T. S., J. DeBoer, and R. L. Persing, Response of wethers to medial lethal dose levels of ^{60}Co gamma radiation, U.S. Air Force Weapons Laboratory, USAFWL-TR-69-145, January (1970).

10. Mobley, T. S., E. T. Still, W. Rush, J. F. Taylor, R. L. Persing, and T. C. DeFeo, Interlaboratory comparison of mortality in sheep exposed to ^{60}Co gamma radiation. U.S. Air Force Weapons Laboratory, USAFWL-TR-69-48, October (1969).

11. Taylor, J. F., E. J. Ainsworth, N. P. Page, and G. F. Leong, Influence of exposure aspect on radiation lethality in sheep. U.S. Naval Radiological Defense Laboratory, USNRDL-TR-69-15, March (1969).

12. Bond, V. P. and C. V. Robinson, A mortality determinant in non-uniform exposures of the mammal. Rad. Res. Suppl. 7: 265-275 (1967).

13. Taylor, J. F., N. P. Page, E. T. Still, G. F. Leong, and E. J. Ainsworth, The effect of exposure rate on radiation lethality in swine. U.S. Naval Radiological Defense Laboratory, USNRDL-TR-69-96, July (1969).

14. Nachtwey, D. S., E. J. Ainsworth, and G. F. Leong, Recovery from radiation injury in swine as evaluated by the split-dose technique. Rad. Res. 31: 353-367 (1967).

15. Brown, D. G. and R. G. Cragle, Some observations of dose-rate effect of radiation on burros, swine, and cattle. In: Dose Rate in Mammalian Biology, D. G. Brown, R. G. Cragle, and T. R. Noonan, eds. pp. 5.1-5.6. USAEC, CONF-680410 (1968).

16. Ainsworth, E. J., G. F. Leong, K. Kendall, and E. L. Alpen, Comparative lethality responses of neutron- and x-irradiated dogs: Influence of dose rate and exposure aspect. Rad. Res. 26: 32-43 (1965).

17. Hauver, R. C., V. T. Penikas, W. J. Walker, M. M. Nold, and T. S. Mobley, Exposure of sheep to millisecond versus microsecond fission radiation. In: Dose Rate in Mammalian Biology, D. G. Brown, R. G. Cragle, and T. R. Noonan, eds. pp. 6.1-6.14. USAEC, CONF-680410 (1968).

18. Mobley, T. S., W. J. Walker, Jr., and J. de Boer, Lethal dose studies on sheep exposed to pulsed fission spectrum radiation (PFSR). U.S. Air Force Weapons Laboratory, USAFWL-TR-65-199, June (1967).

19. Taylor, J. F., E. T. Still, N. P. Page, G. F. Leong, and E. J. Ainsworth, Acute lethality and recovery of goats after 1 MVp x-irradiation. Rad. Res. 45: 110-126 (1971).

20. Taylor, J. F., J. L. Terry, M. E. Ekstrom, and J. E. West, Temporal change in radiosensitivity of miniature swine as evaluated by the split-dose technique. U. S. Armed Forces Radiobiology Research Institute, USAFRRI SR74-14, July (1974).

21. Still, E. T., J. F. Taylor, G. F. Leong, E. J. Ainsworth, Mortality of sheep subjected to acute and subsequent protracted irradiation. U.S. Naval Radiological Defense Laboratory, USNRDL-TR-69-32, June (1969).

22. Hanks, G. E., E. J. Ainsworth, G. F. Leong, D. S. Nachtwey, and N. P. Page, Injury accumulation and recovery in sheep exposed to protracted cobalt-60 gamma radiation. Rad. Res. 29: 211-221 (1966).

23. Page, N. P., E. J. Ainsworth, and G. F. Leong, The relationship of exposure rate and exposure time to radiation injury in sheep. Rad. Res. 33: 94-106 (1968).

24. Page, N. P., E. J. Ainsworth, J. F. Taylor, and G. F. Leong, Recovery of sheep after whole-body irradiation: A comparison of changes in radiosensitivity after acute or protracted exposure. Rad. Res. 46: 301-316 (1971).

Acute Lethality and Radiosensitivity of the Canine Hemopoietic System to Cobalt-60 Gamma and Mixed Neutron-Gamma Irradiation

T.J. MacVittie, R.L. Monroy, M.L. Patchen, and J.H. Darden

Experimental Hematology Department, Armed Forces Radiobiology Research Institute, Bethesda, Maryland 20814, USA

Introduction

Extrapolation of data obtained from model animal systems to predict the human biological response to ionizing radiation and subsequent stressors, such as trauma and/or infectious disease, remains a difficult problem. The choice of animal model is critical in making reliable decisions concerning diagnosis and treatment following single or combined injuries. The canine plays a central role as an appropriate large animal model for extrapolation of the human response to a variety of stressors, whether radiation alone, or in combination with some form of trauma.

The combined injury (CI), where the primary form of energy is exposure to a sublethal dose of ionizing radiation, is a relevant model of study for civilian and defense laboratories. The majority of injuries after a nuclear disaster will be of this type, where two individually sublethal events are transformed into a synergistic lethal response for the combined injured host (27,28). This presents the physician with alternatives not previously encountered, the patient suffering from trauma and also from irradiation. Choice of treatment in some instances must be based not only on the initial condition of the patient, but also on the situation that will exist 7 to 21 days later. In such cases, consideration of total dose, quality of radiation, exposure aspect, and time since exposure are essential (27,28). In the context of the CI program at AFRRI, it is imperative that we describe experimentally the essential features of the radiobiology of our canine model.

This paper will focus on several aspects of the canine hemopoietic response to cobalt-60 gamma (γ) or mixed-fission neutron-gamma (n/γ) radiation, to include (a) lethality, (b) hematological and hemopoietic response and recovery, and (c) estimates of relative biologic effect (RBE).

Materials and Methods

Animals

Healthy, pure-bred, male and female beagles (9-12 kg) were used in these studies. The dogs were treated to eliminate parasitic infections, immunized against distemper, hepatitis, and rabies, and then were observed for 2 weeks before entering the experimental protocol. They were housed in temperature-controlled rooms, in individual stainless steel cages, and were fed kibbled laboratory dog food, supplemented once a week with high-protein, canned meat ration. Water was provided ad libitum.

Hematological values and hemopoietic culture techniques

Peripheral blood was withdrawn from the cephalic vein, and bone marrow was aspirated from the ribs and iliac crest of anesthetized dogs (Biotal, Parke Davis, A.J. Buck & Son, Baltimore, MD) into heparinized syringes. Peripheral blood leukocytes and platelets were counted, using a hemacytometer. Plasma from a 1 ml aliquot of citrated blood was harvested for assay of colony-stimulating activity (CSA). A 5 ml aliquot of citrated blood was used for separation of mononuclear cells (PBMNC), using Lymphocyte Separation Medium (LSM, Bionetics, Kensington, MD) and centrifuged at 1500 rpm (400 x g) for 35 min. The mononuclear cell layer (MNC) was harvested and counted for viable nucleated cells, in a hemocytometer. BM-derived mononuclear cells were harvested in a similar manner. These cell populations were then assayed for specific hemopoietic progenitor cells.

Granulocyte-macrophage (GM-CFC) and macrophage (M-CFC) colony-forming cells were assayed, using the double-layer agar technique previously described (25). Briefly, CSA was provided by using pooled plasma from dogs previously injected with lipopolysaccharide (E. coli, 055:B5, List Biologicals, Campbell, CA) that was added to the bottom agar layer (7% vol/vol) of triplicate culture dishes. BM-derived MNC and PBMNC were plated in the upper agar layer in concentrations depending on previous treatment. Colonies (50 cells) counted after 10 days and 27 days of culture were considered to be derived from GM-CFC and M-CFC, respectively.

Erythroid progenitor cells (CFU-e) were assayed, using the plasma clot technique. For each cell sample, 2 ml of the plasma clot suspension were prepared to contain 0.6 ml heat-inactivated fetal bovine serum, 0.2 ml 25% beef embryo extract, 0.2 ml 10% bovine serum albumin, 0.2 ml (0.04 mg) L-asparagine, 0.2 ml 10^{-3} M 2-mercaptoethanol, 0.2 ml (1 unit) sheep erythropoietin (Step III, Ep, Connaught Medical Research Labs., Swiftwater, PA), 0.2 ml cells (concentrations yielding 1×10^5 to 5×10^6 cells per clot were used), and 0.2 ml 37°C bovine citrated plasma. All ingredients were either reconstituted or diluted, with supplemented alpha medium (SAM) (35), and central plasma clots contained SAM in place of Ep. Immediately, 0.5 ml of this mixture was pipetted into each of three 17-mm flat-bottomed wells in Linbro tissue culture plates, allowed to clot, and incubated for 72 hours at 37°C in humidified atmosphere containing 5% CO_2 in air. Plasma clots were then harvested, fixed with 5% gluteraldehyde, stained with benzidine and geimsa, and scored at 250X using a conventional light microscope.

Cobalt-60 and mixed neutron-gamma irradiation parameters

The beagle dogs were secured in plexiglass holders for both types of exposure. Cobalt-60 irradiation was bilateral at a dose rate of 0.1 Gy per minute to various total-body, midline tissue-absorbed doses (MTD). Mixed neutron-gamma irradiation was achieved in a gadolinium-lined exposure room from the AFRRI TRIGA Mark-F pool-type thermal research reactor, operated in the steady-state mode. Bilateral exposure was 180-degree rotation at midtime of the exposure. The physical parameters of the free-in-air exposure were an average neutron energy of 1.0 MeV and an average gamma energy of 0.9 MeV, a neutron-to-gamma ratio of approximately 6 to 1, and a dose-rate of 0.6 Gy per min. (The neutron to gamma ratio was achieved by imposing a 15 cm-thick lead wall in front of the reactor core tank wall in the exposure room.)

Depth dose measurements were made at the center of a cylindrical phantom (Table 1). The 15.2-cm diameter of the phantom was approximate to the mean 16-cm diameter determined from measurement of 54 dog cadavers. The phantom was made of 0.32 cm lucite and filled with muscle equivalent liquid. The total neutron plus gamma dose measured at phantom midline was 49% of that measured free-in-air; this figure was used to calculate MTD for all dog irradiations. Dose measurements were performed with paired 0.5-cc ion chambers, specifially an A-150 plastic

TABLE 1

Depth Dose Measurements in a Beagle Phantom
and Seven Beagle Cadavers

Comparison of Midline to Free-in-Air Doses	Measured in Phantom	Measured in Cadavers (±1 sigma)
TRIGA Reactor		
Midline neutron dose (% air)	28%	34±(12)%
Midline gamma dose (% air)	210%	206±(21)%
Midline total dose (% air)	49%	52±(11)%
Midline neutron-gamma dose ratio	1.1	1.4±(0.5)
Cobalt-60		
Midline gammma dose (% air)	90%	----

tissue-equivalent chamber with methane-based, tissue-equivalent gas and a magnesium chamber with argon gas. Actual animal irradiations were monitored with ionization chambers and sulfur activation foils mounted at fixed positions in the exposure room to provide corrections for reactor output variations.

Groups of dogs were exposed to MTD's of 1.50 Gy and 2.50 Gy cobalt-60 gamma radiation or 0.75 Gy to 1.25 Gy mixed neutron-gamma irradiation for hemopoietic studies. Additional dogs were exposed to various MTD's of neutron-gamma radiation to determine an LD50(30) value.

Antibiotic, fluid, and platelet therapy

Antibiotics, ampicillin, 500 mg, (Polycillin-N, Bristol Labs, Syracuse, NY) and Gentamycin Sulfate, 30 mg (Garamycin, Schering Pharmaceutical Corp., Kenilworth, NJ) were administered daily until the WBC level reached 1000/mm^3. Fluid support (lactated Ringer's solution) was administered intravenously as dictated by clinical symptoms. Platelets (3-5 x 10^{10}), obtained by plateletpheresis of donor animals, were irradiated with 5,000 rads (cobalt-60 source) and transfused to dogs on days 12, 15, and 18 postirradiation.

Results

Lethality over 30-day period LD50(30) following exposure to mixed neutron-gamma radiation

Shown in Figure 1 are the 30-day mortality values for beagles bilaterally exposed in the AFRRI TRIGA reactor to a range of doses of mixed neutron-gamma radiation. These data would place the LD50(30) value at approximately 1.15 Gy, midline tissue dose for the unsupported dogs. Support in the form of antibiotics, fluids, and platelets can effectively reduce the lethality associated with 1.25 Gy exposure. The

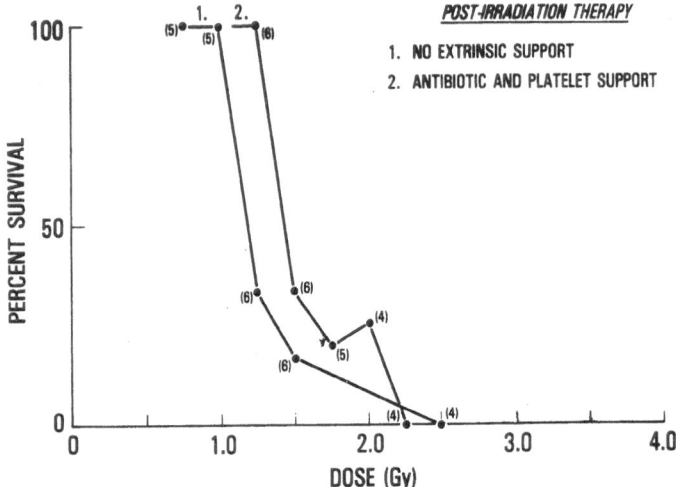

Figure 1. Percent survival of dogs following mixed neutron-gamma whole-body irradiation. (1) No extrinsic support following exposure. (2) Antibiotic and platelet support. Mean values for percent survivors, total dogs at that dose level (n).

TABLE 2

Summary of Literature Values for LD50(30) in Dogs
Exposed to Acute Whole-Body Irradiation

Dogs	Radiation	Dose Rate (R,r/min)	MTD (rads)	Reference
Mongrel	50 kVp	48r	225	Alpen & Baum, A.N.Y.A.S. 114:284(64)
Mongrel	200 kVp	6R	260	Prosser et al., Oak Ridge (56)
Beagle	250 kVp	17r	206	George et al., AFRRI SR68-3 (68)
Mongrel	250 kVp	6R	228	Alpen et al. Radiol. 70:541(58)
Mongrel	250 kVp	15R	252	Bond et al. Rad. Res. 4:139(56)
Mongrel	250 kVp	12R	220	Alpen & Jones, Radiol. 72:81(59)
Mongrel	250 kVp	12r	212	Alpen & Baum, A.N.Y.A.S. 114:284(64)
Beagle	1000 kVp	60R	253	Maille et al., Health Phys. 12:883(66)
Beagle	1000 kVp	50r	250	Hansen et al., Public Health Rep. 76:242(61)
Beagle	1 MVp	10R	288	Earle et al., Rad. Res. 45:487(71)
Mongrel	1 MVp	10R	280	Ainsworth et al., Rad. Res. 26:32(65)
Foxhound	2000 kVp	15R	262	Gleiser, A. J. Vet. Res., 14:284(53)
Mongrel	60Co	30r	260	Wang & Davidson, USAMRL #483 (61)
Beagle	60Co	10-15R	258(AAD)[1]	Norris et al., Rad. Res. 35:681(68)
Mongrel	60Co	6R	335R (301r)[1]	Shively et al., Rad. Res. 9:445(58)
Beagle	60Co	25r	256(AAD)[1]	Garner et al., Rad. Res. 58:190(74)
Beagle	14.6 MeV	2R	281	Earle et al., Rad. Res. 45:487(71)
Mongrel	9 MeV	15R	265	Bond et al., Rad. Res. 4:139(56)
Mongrel	1 MeV	--	239	Alpen et al., Rad. Res. 12:237(60)
Mongrel	1 MeV	--	203	Ainsworth et al., Rad. Res. 26:32(65)
Beagle	1 MeV	60r	110	Monroy et al., this paper
Beagle	n:γ	17r	210	Pitchford & Thorp, AFRRI 68-15 (68)
Beagle	n:γ	17r	218	George et al., AFRRI SR68-3 (68)

[1] Average absorbed dose = AAD, Shively reported dose as midline air dose. Using 0.9 as tissue air ratio for cobalt-60 exposure, the dose is reduced to 268 rads.

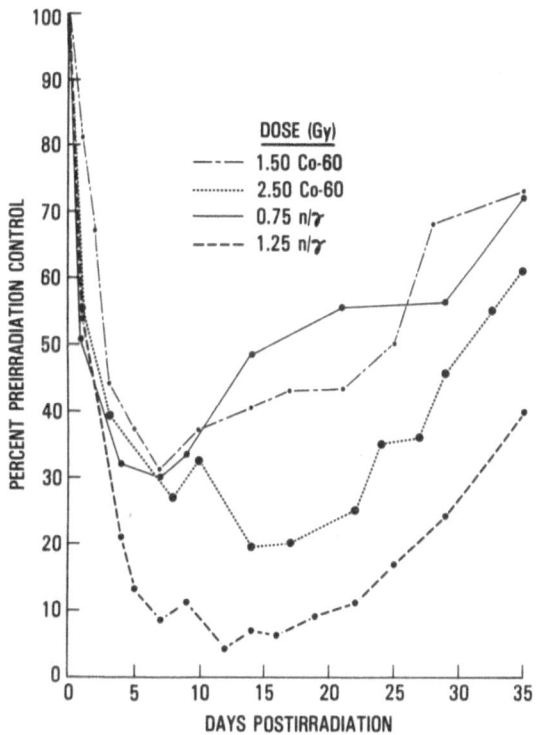

Figure 2. Peripheral blood leukocytes as percent of preirradiation values following exposure to (a) 1.50 Gy cobalt-60 gamma, (b) 2.50 Gy cobalt-60 gamma, (c) 0.75 Gy neutron-gamma and (d) 1.25 Gy neutron-gamma radiation measured as midline tissue absorbed dose. Mean values of 4 to 6 dogs.

effective LD50(30) would be raised to approximately 1.40 Gy of the n/γ exposure. We have not as yet been able to accumulate mortality data for cobalt-60 exposure. However, values in literature (Table 2) place the LD50(30) for cobalt-60 bilateral exposure at approximately 2.60 Gy (15,21,29,34). Thus, based on MTD values, the RBE for hemopoietic lethality would be approximately 2.26.

The MTD chosen for a sublethal exposure to cobalt-60 gamma radiation in our experimental protocol for the Combined Injury Program is 1.50 Gy. An equivalent MTD of mixed neutron-gamma radiation, however, resulted in an approximate LD85(30). This dose had to be reduced to 1.00 Gy before no lethality was observed. Based on an apparent RBE greater than 2.0 using MTD values, the hemopoietic analysis following exposure to mixed neutron-gamma radiation was conducted at a sublethal MTD of 0.75 Gy. Additional analyses were performed after doses of 2.50 Gy gamma and 1.25 mixed neutron-gamma radiation to further illustrate the relative potency or biologic effect of the neutron-gamma exposure.

Peripheral Blood Leukocytes and Platelets

Shown in Figure 2 are the effects of 1.50 Gy and 2.50 Gy gamma radiation relative to 0.75 Gy and 1.25 Gy mixed neutron-gamma radiation on peripheral blood white cells (PBL). Examination of these curves confirms the greater relative potency of neutron-gamma radiation over the cobalt-60 gamma exposure. Each of the two neutron exposures resulted in a more rapid decrease in peripheral white cells when compared to their respective gamma exposures. Peripheral blood leukocytes in the 0.75 Gy neutron exposure reached their nadir sooner (4d) than the 1.50 Gy gamma dogs (7d), although both recovered at the same rate thereafter. The effect of the neutron exposure is more evident at the higher doses where PBL in the 1.25 Gy neutron group reached their nadir within 7-12 d relative to approximately 15 d in the 2.50 Gy gamma group. The neutron exposure also induced a greater decrease in peripheral leukocytes, to about 6% of normal.

TABLE 3

Effect of 1.50 Gy Cobalt-60 Gamma or 0.75 Gy Mixed Neutron:Gamma Radiation on Circulating Platelet Levels[1]

| Time (days) | Platelets (% of Pre-irradiation) | |
	1.50 Gy Gamma	0.75 Gy Neutron:Gamma
Pre-irradiation	100	100
1	90±1.7	100±2.1
3	87±2.0	100±4.8
5	78±3.1	93±4.0
7	75±2.0	80±2.1
10	23±4.1	30±6.7
14	21±1.5	15±3.0
17	19±0.9	15±1.3
21	23±1.7	25±1.7
28	54±8.2	56±6.5
35	93±7.5	75±7.1
42	87±4.4	85±3.4

[1]Mean values (±SEM) of 10 replicate and 5 replicate exposures for 1.50 Gy gamma and 0.75 Gy neutron:gamma exposures respectively.

The decrease in levels of circulating platelets shows a similar effect (Table 3). A dose of 0.75 Gy neutron radiation produced an equivalent hematological effect relative to 1.50 Gy gamma radiation. After both radiation doses, platelet levels decrease slowly during the first week, and then drop precipitously to a nadir of approximately 20% within 10-14 days postexposure. Thereafter, recovery toward normal values proceeds slowly, requiring a total of 5-6 weeks postexposure.

Sensitivity of granulopoietic (GM-CFC) and macrophage (M-CFC) progenitors to cobalt-60 and neutron-gamma radiation

The percent survival of GM-CFC and M-CFC per 10^5 MNC relative to preirradiation values for both types of radiation exposure in the dose range of 0.25 Gy to 3.50 Gy is shown in Figures 3 and 4. The calculation of the dose-response over the exponential portion of the survival curves (semi-log plot) yields the D_0 value.

The respective D_0 values for GM-CFC harvested 24 hours after exposure are approximately 0.73 Gy and 0.30 Gy for cobalt-60 and neutron-gamma radiation, respectively (Figure 3). Calculation of D_0 values for M-CFC yield a similar response, 0.89 Gy and 0.40 Gy for cobalt-60 and mixed neutron-gamma radiation, respectively (Figure 4). These hemopoie-

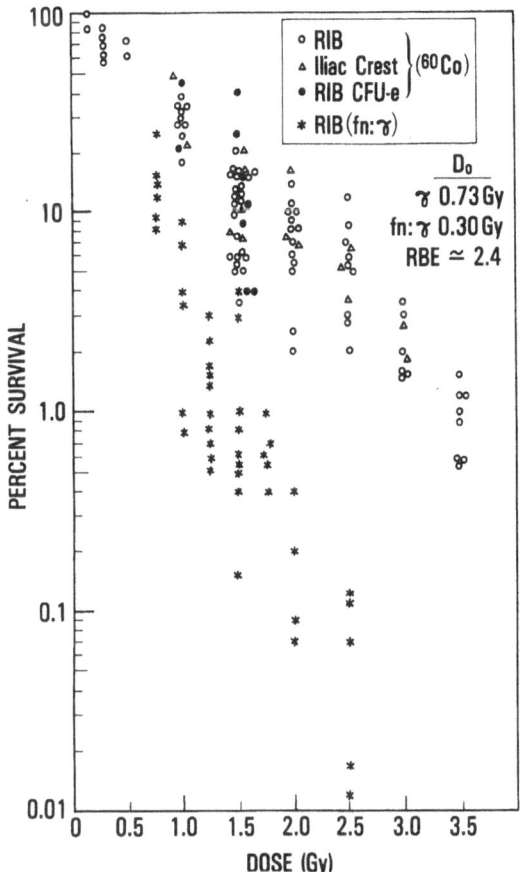

Figure 3. Percent survival of GM-CFC assayed 24 hours postexposure to cobalt-60 gamma or mixed neutron-gamma radiation over the dose (MTD) range of 0.25 Gy to 3.50 Gy.

tic responses are again calculated from midline tissue-absorbed doses. Based on these D_q values, an apparent RBE of greater than 2.0 exists for in vivo sensitivity of GM-CFC and M-CFC to mixed neutron-gamma exposure relative to cobalt-60 gamma exposure. Note that the same total MTD of 1.50 Gy of cobalt-60 or neutron-gamma reduced GM-CFC survival levels to approximately 12% and 0.9%, respectively. Figure 2 also contains values for the response of the erythroid progenitor cell, the CFU-e, to several doses of cobalt-60 gamma radiation. There are inadequate numbers to determine a survival curve but from the values recorded, they appear to lie within the response of the GM-CFC.

Recovery of bone marrow- and peripheral blood-derived GM-CFC following gamma or neutron-gamma irradiation

Recovery of granulopoietic progenitor cells (GM-CFC) was recorded after exposure to 1.50 Gy gamma and 0.75 Gy and 1.25 Gy mixed neutron-gamma irradiation (Figs. 5,6,7). Each recovery curve is characterized by the initial dose-dependent drop in GM-CFC's (Fig. 3). Recovery begins at that point but it depends, of course, on input from a more

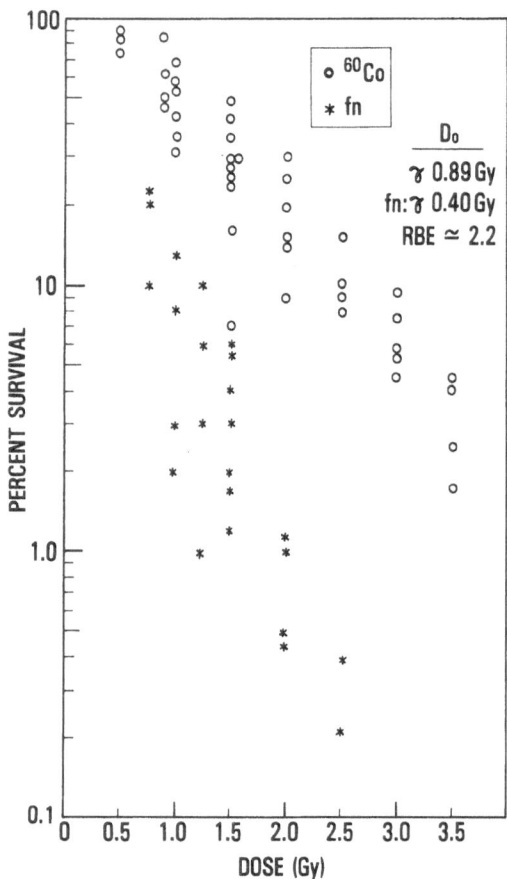

Figure 4. Percent survival of M-CFC assayed 24 hours postexposure to cobalt-60 gamma or mixed neutron-gamma radiation over the dose (MTD) range of 0.25 Gy to 3.50 Gy.

primitive stem cell population that is presumably also affected not only by radiation dose but also by the quality of the radiation. A dose of 1.50 Gy gamma radiation decreased GM-CFC levels to approximately 12% of control. The GM-CFC remained depressed through 5 days. A marked recovery phase followed from day 7 through day 21, after which recovery rate slowed and reached normal levels within 35 days postexposure (Fig. 5). The response of the GM-CFC population to 0.75 Gy neutron-gamma radiation is qualitatively and quantitatively similar to the 1.50 Gy gamma recovery curve, except that complete recovery was extended through 42 days (Fig. 6). The recovery pattern following 1.25 Gy neutron-gamma appears to be much slower and will most likely be extended to 8 or 10 weeks for complete recovery (Fig. 7).

The levels of circulating GM-CFC are significantly more sensitive to 1.50 Gy gamma radiation than the bone marrow-derived GM-CFC (Fig. 8). GM-CFC concentration per 10^5 peripheral blood mononuclear cells are undetectable through 7 days after exposure. They are detected at 10 days and gradually increase in concentration over the next several weeks, but their level remains significantly below preirradiation levels through 6 weeks postirradiation.

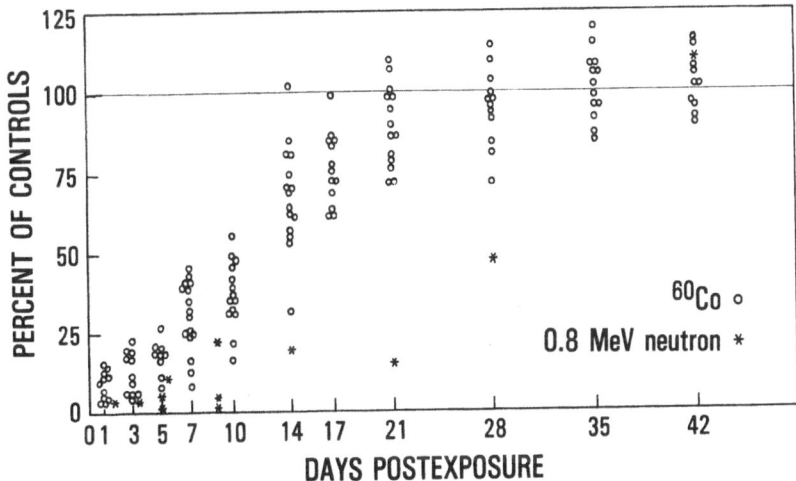

Figure 5. Recovery of bone marrow-derived GM-CFC as percent of pre-irradiation values following exposure to 1.50 Gy gamma radiation. Each value represents individual dog repsonse.

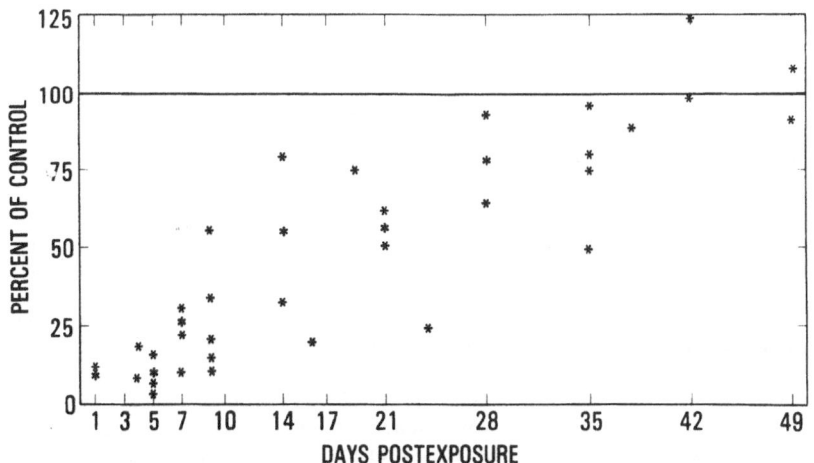

Figure 6. Recovery of bone marrow-derived GM-CFC as percent of pre-irradiation values following exposure to 0.75 Gy mixed neutron-gamma radiation. Each value represents individual dog response.

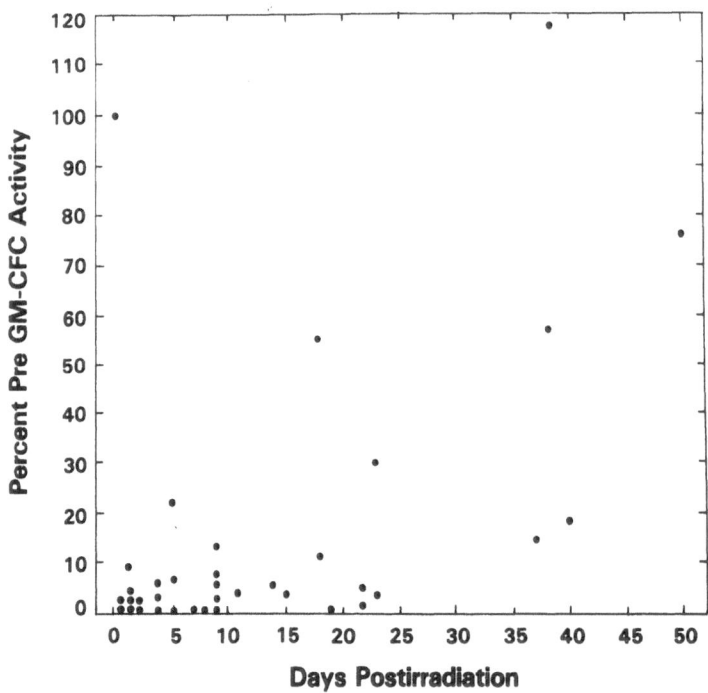

Figure 7. Recovery of bone marrow-derived GM-CFC as percent of pre-irradiation values following exposure to 1.25 Gy mixed neutron-gamma radiation. Each value represents individual dog response.

Discussion

This presentation will describe the canine response to radiations of different quality (that is, cobalt-60 gamma and mixed fission neutron-gamma radiation) in terms of lethality, hematological values, D_o values, hemopoietic recovery, and relative biologic effect.

Lethality and RBE: There is a significant amount of literature that establishes the LD50(30) for hemopoietic death of the canine at approximately 2.60 Gy for cobalt-60 gamma irradiation (15,21,29,34) and X-irradiation of the energies 1000 kVp and 2000 kVp (1,14,18-20) and an average of 2.28 Gy for exposure to lower energy (50-250 kVp) X-irradiation (3-5,7,16,26). These published data indicated a negligible RBE between the cobalt-60 and high energy X-rays but did estimate a small but significant RBE of 0.87 for these higher energy radiations compared to the standard 200-250 kVp X-irradiation. This value is similar to the RBE reported by Sinclair (30) for LD50(30) values in the mouse, relative to gamma and X-irradiation.

Exposure of the beagle to our TRIGA mixed-fission neutron-gamma source resulted in an LD50(30) of 1.15 Gy MTD. This value is significantly lower than LD50(30) MTD values for fission neutrons of the

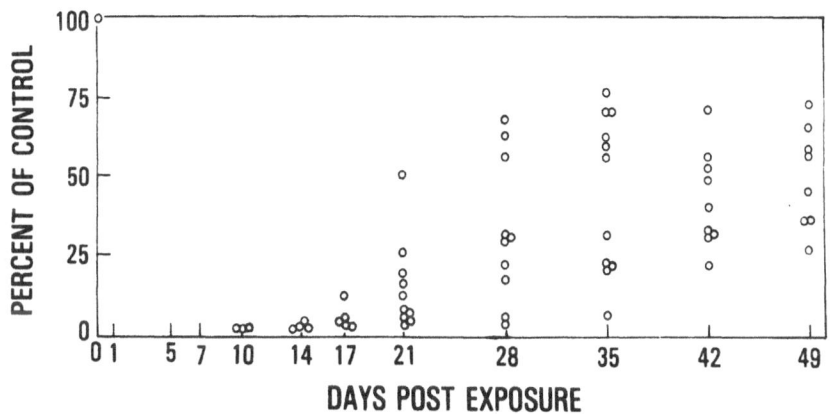

Figure 8. Recovery of peripheral blood-derived GM-CFC as percent of preirradiation values following exposure to 1.50 Gy gamma radiation. Each value represents individual dog response.

comparable 1 MeV energy published by Alpen et al., (6) and Ainsworth et al., (1) of 239 rads and 203 rads, respectively. Calculation of the RBE by these investigators resulted in values of approximately 0.90 for Alpen et al. (6), with reference to 250 kVp X-irradiation and 1.38 for Ainsworth et al. (1), with reference to 1 mVp X-irradiation (Table 4). Our observed RBE relative to the standard 250 kVp X-ray exposure would be approximately 2.0 based on the reported average MTD LD50(30) of 228 rads versus our value of 115 rads, an RBE significantly higher than that previously reported for the canine (Table 4). Table 2 provides a summary of LD50(30) values as MTD for the canine as reported in the literature over approximately the last 20 years. The response to the low LET radiations can be divided into three levels, the 100 to 250 kVp and the 1000 to 2000 kVp X-rays, and the cobalt 60, 1.2 Mev gamma rays. Respective average LD50(30) values are 228 rads, 260 rads, and 268 rads.

TABLE 4

Literature Values for Relative Biologic Effect
of Neutron Exposure versus Gamma or
X-irradiation of LD50(30) Values

Radiation	RBE	Reference
14.6 MeV	1.01	Earle et al.
9.0 MeV	0.95	Bond et al.
1.0 MeV	0.90	Alpen et al.
<1 MeV	1.38	Ainsworth et al.
<1 MeV	1.64	Monroy et al. (unpublished)

Also included in the table are respective LD50(30) values for dogs exposed to neutron radiation of variable energy and mixed neutron-gamma ratios (1,6,7,14,16,24). If our LD50(30) value of 115 rads is compared with that reported for higher energy X-rays or cobalt-60, a greater RBE is observed, based again on MTD. Broerse et al., (10) have reported RBE similar to ours for fission neutrons relative to 1 Mvp X-irradiation in the primate system. They recorded a total absorbed dose of 2.60 Gy for an LD50(30) from fission neutrons of 1 Mev energy relative to 5.25 Gy for 300 kVp X-rays. Thus, the RBE is approximately 2.0 for occurrence of bone marrow lethality in the Rhesus monkey. Stanley et al. (31) and Wise and Turbyfill (38) have also observed a significant RBE in the Rhesus with respect to an LD50(30) end point, utilizing a gamma-neutron exposure versus 250 kVp X-irradiation. Respective MTD values for X-ray and gamma-neutron irradiation were 502 r and 375 r. Similar results have also been observed for LD50(30) values in the murine system. Davids (12,13), Stewart et al., (32), and Ainsworth (2) have all reported RBE values of approximately 2.0 for LD50(30) values for exposure to fission spectrum neutrons, versus cobalt-60 or X-irradiation.

Hemopoietic Response: The 1.50 Gy cobalt-60, whole-body exposure significantly reduced the circulating blood elements, white cells, and platelets as well as the granulopoietic, macrophage, and erythroid progenitor cells. The respective nadirs for peripheral blood leukocytes and platelets were observed at 7 d and 10 d, respectively. These levels remained depressed at approximately 25-35% of preirradiation values through 3 weeks postexposure. Recovery to within normal levels required 5-6 weeks, reflecting the significant but sublethal damage to the marrow stem and progenitor cell pools (17,22,23).

The reason for the depletion of peripheral blood cells is the sensitivity of their respective progenitor cells and the pluripotent stem cell populations to the ionizing radiation. The sensitivity of the canine GM-CFC and M-CFC calculated from survival curves over a broad dose range yield approximate D_o values of 0.73 Gy and 0.89 Gy, respectively. The sensitivity of the GM-CFC population measured as number per 10^5 mononuclear cells is consistent with the literature (9,36). Since we cannot measure the total cellularity of the dog because of experimental design, these values only express the effect of radiation on the relative values of GM-CFC, M-CFC, and CFU-e (per 10^5 MNC) rather than on the absolute number in that marrow location (total per gm of tissue based on total nucleated cells/gm of tissue). Wilson et al. (36), using such a technique for determining absolute recovery of GM-CFC in weanling beagles determined the D_o value to be approximtely 70R following cobalt-60 gamma irradiation. Wilson's results would predict that our 1.50 Gy dose would reduce the rib marrow cellularity to approximately 60% of normal. Since our D_o values are similar (73 rads vs 70R), we could extrapolate our GM-CFC survival fraction to decrease from 12% to roughly 7%, based on total content per gram of rib marrow tissue following 1.50 Gy of gamma radiation.

The RBE based on MTD as observed in our lethality experiments should also be reflected in the radiation sensitivity of marrow progenitor cells, since it is the destruction of these cells that causes the mortality observed during the subsequent 30-day period known as the hemopoietic syndrome. The calculated RBE's for GM-CFC and M-CFC as defined by their D_o values were indeed greater than 2.0 as observed for the LD50(30).

The RBE of approximately 2.0 for low-energy monoenergetic or fission neutrons has also been reported for marrow-derived stem and progenitor cells of the murine and human (9). Boyum et al. (9), using the in vivo diffusion chamber technique for growth of human marrow as well as the GM-CFC technique have shown RBE values of greater than 2.0 versus 250 kVp X-irradiation for neutron energies over the range of 0.44 MeV to 6.0 MeV. The extensive and elegant studies of Ainsworth et al. (2) using the D_q value of murine stem cells as an endpoint and its correlation with LD50(30) values, have shown a consistent RBE or "relative potency" of greater than 2.0. Carsten et al. (11) utilized neutron exposures over the same energy range as Boyum et al. (9) with the D_q values of murine stem cells as an endpoint. They also recorded significant RBE values of greater than 2.0 These laboratories recorded D_q values for exposure to 250 kVp X-irradiation of approximately 80-87 rads versus D_0 values of 28 to 42 rads following exposure to fission spectrum neutrons or of neutrons less than 5 Mev.

The equivalent biological effect may be viewed from another angle. The respective LD50(30)'s for gamma (2.60 Gy) and neutron-gamma (1.15 Gy) should result in a similar percentage survival of marrow progenitor cells. If the bone marrow is indeed the critical target organ, then the stem and progenitor cells residing within the marrow must be target cells. The response of these cells in terms of lethality and recovery should correlate with the LD50(30). Indeed, the observed value taken from the respective survival dose-response curves for GM-CFC at the LD50(30) levels for both gamma and neutron-gamma exposure are approximately 2% survival. We are not saying that the GM-CFC is a stem cell. The GM-CFC is an important progenitor cell, more highly differentiated than the stem cell, but with a similar radiosensitivity in the murine system. If this is valid number and 10^{-2} is a critical surviving fraction in the canine, it is considerably higher than the surviving fractions of between 10^{-3} and 10^{-4} noted for the murine system (2,12,13) where an assay for the stem cell exists.

Ainsworth (2) and Davids (12,13) found a correspondence between the RBE for surviving fractions of stem cells at LD50(30) for fission spectrum neutrons. Ainsworth does indicate that use of the surviving fraction following 250 kVp X-irradiation to calculate the LD50(30) for fission spectrum neutron will result in an underestimate of the dose required, although significant correspondence is observed. It must also be noted that the RBE for the stem cell survival at these dose levels is based on extrapolation.

The final aspect of this report is the recovery time necessary for the marrow granulopoietic progenitor cell levels to return to preirradiation levels. Similar patterns of recovery were observed for the respective 1.50 Gy and 0.75 Gy gamma and neutron-gamma exposures. This is consistent with the "relative potency" of the neutron-gamma exposure as indicated by lethality, dose-response curves, and hematologic response. A similar correlation of these parameters has also been observed in the mouse hemopoietic response to fission neutrons versus 250 kVp X-irradiation (2). The response and recovery of the GM-CFC population to the 1.50 Gy gamma exposure agrees well with the results of Gerhartz et al. (17) and Nothdurft and Fliedner (22,23). These collaborators have performed an extensive series of experiments defining the canine hemopoietic response to a range of sublethal doses of low-energy (300 kVp) X-irradiation. Our data describing the canine response in terms of lethality (LD50(30)), hematologic values, dose-response curves for GM-CFC, and hemopoietic recovery to cobalt-60 gamma and mixed fission neutron-gamma radiation suggest a significant RBE or "relative potency" for the fission spectrum neutron radiation. These results, however, are based on midline tissue-absorbed dose. The MTD was established by Bond et al., (8) to be used as a relevant reference dose, because free-in-air, entrance, and exit doses have not been acceptable substitutes. It was their intent to use a value that would represent the "dose" received by an animal. This value, MTD, was suggested with full recognition that, in irradiating an animal of any size, particularly a dog, some degree of inhomogeneity of dose throughout the tissues will exist, no matter what type of radiation is employed. In quoting a single value for the "dose" received by the animal it is necessary to settle on the dose received at some fixed location within the animal. Bond (7,8) states that the ideal would be to measure the dose received by a specific critical organ that would correlate with the biological endpoint, such as the dose received by the bone marrow in the LD50(30) range. This cannot be done, expecially with reference to neutron and mixed neutron-gamma radiation. In our particular circumstance, we recognize that a complex dosimetric condition exists (Table 1). Our TRIGA exposure of the canine starts with a 6:1 neutron-gamma ratio, free-in-air, with an average neutron energy between 0.8 and 1.0 MeV, and dissipates to a 1:1 ratio at midline, of unknown neutron energy. We do not know (a) the depth dose response, (b) the absorbed dose to the critical organ (the bone marrow), (c) the spectral changes (neutron energy) as the dose is absorbed, and (d) resultant change in neutron-gamma ratio with tissue interaction.

There are, however, two technical reports (33,37) that describe the depth dose within canine and pig cadavers and phantoms from mixed fission neutron-gamma radiation delivered by a TRIGA Mark F reactor. Considering the reactor identity, the approximate body size of the beagle and miniature pig used (approximately 16 cm width, 8 cm midline), the similar neutron-gamma field, and the published depth dose curves taken as percent of total neutron-gamma surface dose, we take the liberty of calculating the total dose delivered to the dog at approximately 3 cm depth. The 3 cm depth is based on the proposed location of a large percentage of active bone marrow.

Radiation	Biological Effect	MTD(Gy)	TAR	FIA Dose Surface (Gy)	3cm Depth Dose %FIA	3cm Depth Dose (Gy)
n/γ	1%S GM-CFC	1.50	0.49	3.06	75%	2.30
γ	1%S GM-CFC	3.56	0.90	3.96	95%	3.76
RBE		2.37				1.64

These calculations reduce the RBE from 2.37 based on MTD to 1.64 based on extrapolation, using Wingates' (37) and Verreli's (33) depth-dose data. The 1.6 value is still considerably higher than the value of 1.38 previously reported by Ainsworth et al. (1) using the same reactor that Wingate evaluted for depth-dose patterns. Ainsworth (2) reported almost 20 years ago that "... it is clear that at present we are unable to accurately measure and partition radiation responses in those cellular systems critical to survival of the neutron-irradiated mouse." We have not progressed very far, especially with regard to the larger animal species. Perhaps it is time that we ask the dosimetry to catch up with the culture techniques. The continued progress in both areas may give us some long-awaited answers.

References

1. Ainsworth, E.J., Leong, G.F., Kendall, K., and Alpen, E.L. Comparative lethality responses of neutron- and X-irradiated dogs: Influence of dose-rate and exposure aspect. Radiat. Res. 26:32-43 (1965).

2. Ainsworth, E.J., Larsen, R.M., Kendall, K., Leong, G.F., Krebs, J.S., and Mitchell, F.A. Recovery in the mouse after neutron-irradiation: Evaluation of injury and recovery using split-dose lethality and repopulation of colony-forming units. Unpublished results (1970).

3. Alpen, E.L. and Baum, S.J. Comparative effects of 50 kVp and 250 kVp X- rays on the dog. Ann. N. Y. Acad. Sci. 114:284-294 (1964).

4. Alpen, E.L. and Jones, D.M. The effects of concomitant superficial X-irradiation upon the lethal effectiveness of 250 kVp X-rays. Radiology 72:81 (1959).

5. Alpen, E.L., Jones, D.M., Hechter, H.H., and Bond, V.P. The comparative biological response of dogs to 250 kVp X-rays and 100 kVp X-rays. Radiology 70:541-549 (1958).

6. Alpen, E.L., Shill, O.S., and Tochilin, E. The effects of total body irradiation of dogs with simulated fission neutrons. Radiat. Res. 12:237-250 (1960).

7. Bond, V.P., Carter, R.E., Robertson, J.S., Seymour, P.H., and Hechter, H.H. The effects of total-body fast neutron irradiation in dogs. Radiat. Res. 4:139-153 (1956).

8. Bond, V.P., Cronkite, E.P., Sondhaus, C.A., Imirie, G., Robertson, J.S., and Borg, D.C. The influence of exposure geometry on the pattern of radiation dose delivered to large animal phantoms. Radiat. Res. 6:554-563 (1957).

9. Boyum, A., Carsten, A.L., Chikkappa, G., Cook, L., Bullis, J., Honikel, L., and Cronkite, E.P. The r.b.e. of different-energy neutrons as determined by human bone-marrow cell culture techniques. Int. J. Radiat. Biol. 34:201-212 (1978).

10. Broerse, J.J., van Bekkum, D.W., Hollander, C.F., and Davids, J.A.G. Mortality of monkeys after exposure to fission neutrons and the effect of autologous bone marrow transplantation. Int. J. Radiat. Biol. 34:253-264 (1978).

11. Carsten, A.L., Bond, V.P., and Thompson, K. The r.b.e. of different energy neutrons as measured by the haematopoietic spleen-colony technique. Int. J. Radiat. Biol. 29:65-70 (1976).

12. Davids, J.A.G. Relative biological effectiveness of fission neutrons for production of the bone marrow syndrome in mice. Int. J. Radiat. Biol. 10:299-310 (1966).

128

13. Davids, J.A.G. Acute effects of 1 Mev fast neutrons on the haemo-poietic tissues, intestinal epithelium and gastric epithelium in mice. Advances in Radiation Research, Volume 2, pp 565-576 (1970).

14. Earle, J.D., Ainsworth, J.E., and Leong, G.F. Lethal and hemato-logic effects of 14.6 Mev neutrons on beagles with estimation of RBE. Radiat. Res. 45:487-498 (1971).

15. Garner, R.J., Phemister, R.D., Angleton, G.M., Lee, A.C., and Thomassen, R.W. Effect of age on the acute lethal response of the beagle to cobalt-60 gamma radiation. Radiat. Res. 58:190-195 (1974).

16. George, R.E., Stanley, R.E., Wise, D., and Barron, E.L. The acute mortality response of beagles to mixed gamma-neutron radiations and 250 kVp X-rays. Armed Forces Radiobiology Research Institute SR 68-3 (1968).

17. Gerhartz, H.H., Nothdurft, W., and Fliedner, T.M. Effect of low dose whole-body irradiation on granulopoietic progenitor cell sub-populations: Implications for CFUc release. Cell Tissue Kinet. 15:371-379 (1982).

18. Gleiser, C.A. The determination of the lethal dose 50/30 of total body X-irradiation for dogs. Am. J. Vet. Res. 14:284-286 (1953).

19. Hansen, C.L., Michaelson, S.M., Howland, S.W. Lethality of upper body exposure n in beagles. Public Health Rep. 76:242-246 (1961).

20. Maille, H.D., Krasavage, W., and Mermagen, H. On the partial-body irradiation of the dog. Health Physics 12:883-887 (1966).

21. Norris, W.P., Fritz, T.E., Rehfeld, C.E., and Poole, C.M. The response of the beagle dog to cobalt-60 gamma radiation: Deter-mination of the LD50(30) and description of associated changes. Radiat. Res. 35:681-708 (1968).

22. Nothdurft, W., and Fliedner, T.M. The response of the granulocytic progenitor cells (CFU-c) of blood and bone marrow in dogs exposed to low doses of X-irradiation. Radiat. Res. 89:38-52 (1982).

23. Nothdurft, W., Steinbach, K.H., and Fliedner, T.M. In vitro studies on the sensitivity of canine granulopoietic progenitor cells (GM-CFC) to ionizing radiation. Differences between steady state GM-CFC from blood and bone marrow. Int. J. Radiat. Biol. 43:133-140 (1983).

24. Pitchford, T.L. and Thorp, J.W. The acute mortality response of beagles to pulsed mixed gamma-neutron radiations. Armed Forces Radiobiology Research Institute SR 68-15 (1968).

25. Porvaznik, M. and MacVittie, T.J. Detection of gap junctions be-tween the progeny of a canine macrophage colony-forming cell in vitro. J. Cell. Biol. 82:555-564 (1979).

26. Prosser, C.L., Painter, E.E., and Swift, M.N. In: Biological Effects of External X- and Gamma Radiation (ed. Zirkle, R.E.), part 2, pp. 1-99, U.S. Atomic Energy Commission, Technical Information Service Extension. Oak Ridge, TN, JID 5220 (1956).

27. Schraiber, M.I. and Korchanov, L.S. Relevance of radiation injury in the combined injury syndrome. Intermedes Proceedings. Combined injuries and Shock. (eds. B. Schildt, L. Thoren) pp. 17-20 (1968).

28. Schildt, B., and Thoren, L. Experimental and clinical aspects of combined injuries. Intermedes Proceedings. Combined Injuries and Shock (eds. Schildt, B. and Thoren, L.) (1968).

29. Shively, J.N., Michaelson, S.M., and Howland, J.W. The response of dogs to bilateral whole-body cobalt-60 irradiation. I. Lethal dose determination. Radiat. Res. 9:445-450 (1958).

30. Sinclair, W.K. The relative biological effectiveness of 22-Mevp X-rays, cobalt-60 gamma rays, and 200-kvcp X-rays. VII. Summary of studies for five criteria of effect. Radiat. Res. 16:394-398 (1962).

31. Stanley, R.E., Seigneur, L.J., and Strike, T.A. The acute mortality response of monkeys (Macaco Mulatta) to mixed gamma-neutron radiations and 250 kVp X-rays. Armed Forces Radiobiology Research Institute SR66-23 (1966).

32. Stewart, D.A., Ledney, G.D., Baker, W.H., Daxon, E.G., and Sheehy, P.A. Bone marrow transplantation of mice exposed to a modified fission neutron (N/G-30:1) field. Radiat. Res. 92:268-279 (1982).

33. Verrelli, D.M. and Shosa, D.W. Comparison of dose patterns in a miniature pig exposed to neutron and to gamma radiation. Armed Forces Radiobiology Reserch Institute, TN 71-5, Oct. 1971.

34. Wang, R.I.H. and Davidson, D.E., Jr. Experimental conditions for acute whole-body irradiation of dogs with cobalt-60. U.S. Army Medical Research Laboratory Report No. 483 (1961).

35. Weinberg, S.R., McCarthy, E.G., MacVittie, T.J., and Baum, S.J. Effect of low dose irradiation on pregnant mouse hemopoiesis. Br. J. Haematol. 48:127-135 (1981).

36. Wilson, F.D., Stitzel, K.A., Klein, A.K., Shifrine, M., Graham, R., Jones, M ., Bradley, E., and Rosenblatt, L.S. Quantitative response of bone marrow colony-forming units (CFU-c & PFU-c) in weanling beagles exposed to acute whole-body gamma-irradiation. Radiat. Res. 74:289-297.

37. Wingate, C.L., Page, N.P., and Ainsworth, E.J. Comparison of dose patterns in a dog exposed to neutrons and to X-rays. U.S. Naval Radiological Defense Laboratory, USNRDL-TR-974, Feb, 1966.

38. Wise, D. and Turbyfill, C.L. The acute mortality response of monkeys (Macaco mulatta) to pulsed mixed gamma-neutron radiation. Armed Forces Radiobiology Research Institute SR68-17.

SUMMARY OF THE DISCUSSION ON PHYSICAL ASPECTS AND
ACUTE LETHALITY IN DIFFERENT SPECIES

H. Smith

National Radiological Protection Board, Chilton, Didcot, United Kingdom.

As an introduction to the workshop, Broerse reminded participants to the major studies performed in the 1950's and 60's to derive dose-response relationships for acute responses to ionizing radiations. There was now a need to re-examine these data with a view to comparing exposure conditions and to measuring biological endpoints other than death. This was particularly important in providing a scientific basis for clinical studies involving total body irradiations (TBI) followed by bone marrow transplantation. He stressed the need for standardized procedures in patients if the various centres using TBI wished to compare their results in terms of successful destruction of bone marrow cells and recovery following the injection of compatible donor cells.

The session chairman, Silini, indicated that the recommmendations of the workshop would be useful to the secretariat of UNSCEAR, who are in the process of preparing a technical annex on the acute effects of ionizing radiations.

With regard to the presentation by Zoetelief, Fliedner enquired as to the dose variations that might occur in the tissues of patients exposed to high energy radiations from linear accelarators. In reply, Zoetelief referred to studies in phantoms using 4 MV X rays which he felt were applicable to other high energy radiations. Variations of dose in small phantoms (40 cm³) were within the criteria defined by the ICRU (Quantitative concepts and dosimetry in radiobiology, ICRU report 30, 1979) for uniform irradiation, but he admitted that this was not so for dog-sized phantoms. Under these circumstances, bilateral irradiation would be necessary to ensure uniformity of dose throughout the body. In reply to a question from Young, Zoetelief considered that on balance cylindrical phantoms rather than rectangular shaped phantoms were more representative of the dose distribution in the animal, if only data on phantoms were available; but that in addition, scattter and attenuation must be taken into account. In practice it was much better to prepare an animal phantom of tissue equivalent material for reference purposes.

Carsten referred to a chemical tissue equivalent dosemeter embedded in wax which had been used successfully some years ago to measure dose-depth distribution in monkey head phantoms. The wax phantom was sectioned and radiation-induced colour changes measured using a reflecting colour densitometer. He thought that a reproducibility of 5% should be possible with the more sensitive instrumentation now available. This procedure is an improvement on liquid chemical dosemeters which provide only a measure of mean dose.

In connection with his presentation Kaul indicated that he could readjust his model to take account of different marrow distributions according to individual dimensions and further he could give an idea of the sensitivity of the model to these changes. Ainsworth reminded Kaul that the model could be tested by using available experimental data on miniature pigs and dogs exposed in various positions.

Carsten wondered how it was possible to relate neutron to gamma deposition in bone marrow which has a different cross section for these radiations compared to tissue equivalent material and which produces non-uniformly in the skeleton. Kaul replied that Eckerman of Oak Ridge, using Spiers' original methodology applied to human trabecular bone structure, was recalculating dose distribution in the marrow of the Japanese atom bomb victims. He felt that this approach overcame the problems referred to by Carsten, since the dosimetry was standardized on neutron particle fluence and this was relatable to biologically meaningful data in contrast to physical parameters such as kerma and LET.

Ainsworth wondered if Kaul's model included the possibility that death could be due to gastro-intestinal damage after exposure to several gray, despite the prediction that sufficient bone marrow stem cells had survived to ensure recovery from haematopoietic depression. Kaul accepted that gastro-intestinal damage could kill the individual if the dose to the gut exceeded about 15 Gy, even though sufficient marrow was shielded - but reference was not made to an effect at lower doses.

Fliedner was concerned about any model which related marrow cell damage to acute mortality but which did not consider recovery of stem cells and how this recovery may be influenced by the micro-environment of the stem cells. Carsten reminded participants of the work of Werts, Johnson and de Gowin (Radiation Research, $\underline{71}$, 214-224, 1977) where it was shown that irradiation of the bone marrow stroma in rodents to about 10 Gy did not inhibit stromal cell repopulation but inhibition did occur in the region of 50 Gy. These data may be applicable to Kaul's model but it is difficult to see how these murine results can be extrapolated to the human situation.

In reply Kaul accepted these points and emphasized that modelling relating neutral particle fluence to a biological endpoint could accommodate additional data on regeneration capability as this becomes available.

Broerse mentioned that the studies on mice performed at TNO have demonstrated D_0 values of 0.7 Gy and enquired about the effect of changes in the assumed D_0 of the bone marrow stem cell and predictions about human survival. In reply, Kaul stated that changes in D_0 (e.g., from 0.9 to 0.8 Gy) marginally altered this relationship (i.e., a bone marrow stem cell survival of about 10% instead of 13% corresponded to an LD_{50} dose); but these predictions applied to the average man with a normal gut micro-flora. He agreed that survival seemed possible in a carefully prepared patient who received about 0.1% of the normal number of his bone marrow stem cells. He stressed, however, that the real value of his model was to indicate differences between partial body irradiations, the effect of changes in field orientation and of different ratios of neutrons to gamma radiations rather than to relate chances of survival to an absolute fraction of bone marrow stem cells.

In the discussion on Vriesendorp's presentation Carsten offered an alternative explanation as to why young animals are more sensitive to ionizing radiation than adults. It is that the pituitary-hypothalmus-adrenal system is not developed in very young animals and they cannot adapt to the stress of exposure to ionizing radiation as readily as animals with a functional endocrine system.

Fliedner pointed out that in dogs, he had been able to separate out a CFU-c stem cell sub-population from bone marrow which is present in blood. This fraction had a greater ability to repopulate bone marrow than other fractions. He mentioned that cells in this particular fraction, with a D_0 of 0.25 Gy compared to a D_0 of 0.8 Gy for mixed CFU-c bone marrow cells approximated to the pluripotent cell. Vriesendorp, in reply, thought that this cell fraction had little influence upon the animal's survival as the cells found in blood occurred at a concentration of about 1/100th of that in the bone marrow. Fliedner maintained nevertheless that these fractions contained the cells essential to survival, the other fractions containing sub-populations of partially differentiated cells.

In reply to a question from Smith, Vriesendorp indicated that the fraction of surviving stem cells was not the important factor in animal or human survival. It was rather a reduction to a critical number of bone marrow stem cells in the irradiated host. Thus in species with a low number of bone marrow cells it takes less radiation to reduce the number to a critical level. With regard to the importance of bone marrow transplantation, gut sterilisation, blood cell and fluid replacement in influencing the survival of large animals and man, he predicted that such treatment could enhance the LD_{50} by about 1 Gy compared to non-treated animals or individuals.

Van Bekkum added that some animals would die irrespective of the number of bone marrow stem cells injected and the antibiotic treatment used. This was because of resistant micro-organisms. Thus when considering the human, it was impossible to predict the outcome of an infection without knowing the sensitivity of the microbial contaminant to antibiotic treatment.

Following up the comment of Carsten in his prediction that cardio-vascular collapse following haemorrhage plays an important part in influencing survival after a uniform exposure to a few gray of low LET radiation, Kaul reminded participants of the group of 159 farmworkers at Hiroshima who were exposed at a distance of 1000 m from the epicentre of the bomb. The dose to bone marrow in each individual was estimated to be about 2 Gy and just over half the group died within a month of exposure. Anaemia and malnutrition may well have influenced their chances of recovery. Fliedner agreed and added that severe anaemia following haemorrhage was not a cause of death in fit men accidentally exposed to radiation because they received blood transfusions to correct the blood loss. Nevertheless non-thrombopenic haemorrhage associated with capillary wall damage is commonly seen in experimental animals exposed to mid-lethal doses and it is likely that this situation applies to man.

MacVittie and Conklin indicated that secondary trauma and stress could also influence LD_{50} and they were not surprised at the proposed low LD_{50} at Hiroshima and Nagasaki in view of the circumstances of the exposure.

Silini thanked Ainsworth for presenting some data that had not been previously available in the open literature. He proposed that a measure of recovery rather than lethality was more meaningful as a biological endpoint. Fliedner agreed, indicating that the determinants of lethality were trombocytopenia and granulocytopenia, that the course of development of these blood cell deficiencies was different between species and LD_{50} did not reveal these differences in kinetics. Regeneration and repair of stem cell population would seem to be a more appropriate index of recovery, but a suitable assay had still to be developed.

Ainsworth reminded participants that there was a vast amount of haematological and other clinical data collected from the US large animal studies which were still to be analysed. Critical evaluation of these data may provide insight into the kinetics of blood cell recovery.

Concerning MacVittie's presentation Fliedner wondered why dogs, exposed to 2 Gy and given autologous marrow, platelets, antibiotics and fluid replacement, should die while their bone marrow was regenerating. MacVittie pointed out that the animals were exposed to mixed neutron-gamma radiations and that death was due to gut damage 7-9 days after exposure. He was not in a position to give details of the fluid replacement regime used to maintain these animals.

A general discussion developed about the most appropriate bone marrow colony-forming cell to relate to recovery. The bone marrow GM-CFU cell was not considered to be a good indicator of the pluripotent cells which Van Bekkum claimed he had identified in the mouse. This was the cell of choice. Fliedner on the other hand, had fractionated a sub-population of cells from bone marrow of the dog which was similar in regenerative capacity to cells found in blood. He maintained that this sub-population approximated to the pluripotent cell. It is clear that the elusive pluripotent cell has yet to be positively identified in large animals and man.

Silini questioned the need to use large experimental animals to characterize mechanisms of haematopoiesis after exposure to ionizing radiations. MacVittie and Conklin pointed out that the rodent could not be used in place of the dog to provide details of depth-dose distribution of neutrons; or of bone marrow cell kinetics which were species specific; or measuring the RBE of neutrons for gastro-intestinal damage.

Smith asked how pertinent gastro-intestinal damage was in the irradiated human. Fliedner replied that it may be an important contributor to death in the untreated individual at doses greater than several gray of low LET radiation; but that is was not normally seen in patients receiving marrow transplants after TBI because their gut was decontaminated before irradiation and they received adequate fluid replacement during the critical phase of mucosal cell regeneration.

SURVIVAL PATTERNS AND HEMOPATHOLOGICAL RESPONSES OF DOGS UNDER CONTINUOUS
GAMMA IRRADIATION

TM Seed, TE Fritz, DV Tolle, CM Poole, LS Lombard, DE Doyle, LV Kaspar,
SM Cullen, and BA Carnes.
Division of Biological and Medical Research, Argonne National Laboratory,
Argonne, IL, 60439, USA

ABSTRACT

Survival curves were constructed and analyzed relative to contributing
hematopathological responses for groups of beagles exposed continuously
for duration of life to low daily doses of whole body ^{60}Co gamma irradiation (27.3 rads/day to 4 rads/day). The survival curves versus time were
progressively displaced toward longer survival as rates of exposure were
reduced from the relatively high dose rate of 27.3 rads/day to the low
dose rate of 4.0 rads/day. Average survival times increased from 57 days
at 27.3 rads/day to 1830 days at 4.0 rads/day, representing fractional
increased life-spans from 1.5% to 50.8%, respectively. Survival curves
versus total dose were markedly displaced along the cumulative radiation
dose axis at the extreme dose rates (i.e., 27.3 and 4.0 rads/day), but
not at the intermediate dose rates (i.e., 13.4 and 7.9 rads/day) in which
the upper linear portions of the survival curves are superimposed. From
these dose-dependent survival curves, LD_{50} values for whole body gamma
irradiation, delivered chronically at 27.3, 13.4, 7.9, and 4.0 rads per
day were estimated to be 1442, 2124, 2039, and 7161 rads, respectively.
Both time- and dose-dependent survival curves for the intermediate dose
rates, in contrast to the extreme dose rates, exhibited pronounced transitions in the lethality rate below the 50% survival level. These
lethality rate transitions occurred at ~ 2500 rads of accumulated dose
and were attributed to a shift in the spectrum of developing hematopathologies: namely, from a predominance of the acutely ablative radiation-
induced lymphohematopoietic syndromes (i.e., septicemias and aplastic
anemias) to a predominance of the late arising hematopoietic neoplasias
(myelogenous leukemia and related myeloproliferative disorders). Based
on the concept that these lethality rate transitions and shifts in the
spectrum of developing pathologies reflect distinct subgroups of dogs of
varying radiosensitivities and pathological tendencies, estimates of LD_{50}
values for subgroups with specific pathologies are given (e.g., 1850 rads
for the subgroup with aplasia; 5500 rads for the subgroup with myeloproliferative diseases). Sequential analyses of blood and marrow responses
indicated that this shift in hematopathologic spectrum (and in turn the
lethality rate transition) is due to an early reparative hematological
event that is prerequisite to prolonged survival and, in turn, to the
expression of late arising neoplasias. The cellular basis of this repair
appears to be mediated, in part, by an acquisition of radioresistance by
early hematopoietic progenitors.

INTRODUCTION

The hemopathological responses under continuous whole body gamma irradiation and their effect on lethality rates have been extensively studied in small short lived rodents (Lamerton et al., 1960; Twentyman and Blackett, 1970; Pontifex and Lamerton, 1960; Bustad et al., 1965; Lord, 1964, 1965; Blackett, 1967; Kalina and Praslicka, 1977; and Sacher, 1955). The classic studies carried out more than two decades ago by Lamerton and his colleagues demonstrated the relationships among decrementing dose rates, hematopoietic sparing, and incrementing survival times (Lamerton et al., 1960). Sacher and colleagues (1978) analyzed dose rate effects on life shortening for some fifteen different species of mammals from three different orders (i.e., Carnivora, Artiodactyla, and Rodentia). This analysis resulted in the development of a generic lethality/dose rate relation: at very low dose rates, the lethality rate is dependent solely on total cumulative dose and independent of dose rate; at intermediate dose rates, and extending into the higher rates of exposure, the rate of lethality becomes dose-rate dependent. Interestingly, the point of transition (i.e., from dose rate independent to dependent) is apparently a stable characteristic of the species.

In contrast to the rather extensive studies made using small mammals, there is a sparcity of information concerning lethality and hematological response in larger, relatively long-lived species (e.g., dogs) under chronic gamma irradiation, especially at very low rates of exposure. Page et al. (1968) reported that for male western sheep the lethality rate decremented linearly as the rate of gamma ray exposure was reduced from 660 to 30 R/hr, representing an effective increase in the LD_{50}'s from 237 R at 660 R/hr to 338 R at 30 R/hr. At exposure rates below 30 R/hr, lower lethality rates and much higher LD_{50} values (e.g., LD_{50} of 495 R at 3.6 R/hr and 637 R at 2.0 R/hr) were observed. Similar lethality/dose rate relationships have been reported for swine (Brown and Cragle, 1968).

Previously, we had reported LD_{50}'s for chronic, low daily dose gamma radiation using beagles exposed for preset total exposure levels (600-4000 R) rather than for duration of life, as is the case for dogs described in this report (Fritz et al., 1978). Despite this difference in radiation protocol, our estimates from the two approaches are reasonably close, differing by 2-32% at the various dose rates tested.

All of the above large animal studies have suffered from the fact that dose rate effects have been assessed in terms of daily or cumulatively delivered air dose (in roentgens) rather than as an individualized absorbed dose (in rads).

Accordingly, this paper has three objectives: (i) to give our current estimates, based on refined data, of the LD_{50}'s for whole body 60-cobalt gamma radiation delivered chronically to beagles at average daily rates of 35 R (27.3 rads) to 5 R (4.0 rads) per day; (ii) to illustrate the time course for development of the major pathologies responsible for the noted lethality patterns; and finally (iii) to examine a prominent reparative hematopoietic event that appears responsible for marked transitions in rates of lethality and in the spectrum of developing pathologies.

MATERIALS and METHODS

Animals

Outbred beagles included in this study were derived from the closed
Argonne National Laboratory colony whose status, origin, and general
management have been described in detail elsewhere (Norris et al.,
1968). The two hundred and sixteen purebred beagles included in this
study are part of a long range project whose overall aim is to evaluate
morbidity and mortality rates as a consequence of chronically delivered,
whole body gamma irradiation in a relatively large and long lived species
of mammal (Norris and Fritz, 1972; Fritz et al., 1978, 1982). All dogs
were approximately 400 days old at the start of the experiment, anatomi-
cally normal, and in good health. Both male and female animals, at approximately 1/1 ratios, were used in the various groups. The size (chest
dimensions) and weight of experimental animals at the start of the experiment were 14.1 cm (± 1.8 cm, S.D.) and 10.4 kg (± 3.1 kg, S.D.), respectively. Prior to and during the experiment, the test and control dogs
were regularly monitored clinically and hematologically.

Irradiation of Animals

Experimental dogs were maintained in two-tiered standard size fiberglass
cages (71 x 71 x 61 cm) within a specially designed irradiation facility
equipped with an attenuated 9 Ci ^{60}Co source having an effective energy
of approximately 1.0 MeV (Gammabeam-150, Atomic Energy of Canada, Ltd.,
Ottawa). The dog cages were rotated 90° each day and the dogs were moved
from the top tier to the bottom and vice versa once each week in an effort to maximize the uniformity of the air dose delivered to the caged
animals. Dogs were continuously irradiated for duration of life, at
daily exposure rates (measured at the midpoint of the cage) of either 5,
10, 17, or 35 R per 22-hour day (Williamson et al., 1968). During the 2
hours when the dogs were not exposed, they were fed, watered, and clinically manipulated for blood and marrow sample collection. Control animals were similarly treated and handled, except they were maintained
either in cages in a shielded, adjoining anteroom (experimental controls)
or in standard pens (colony controls). The responses of the chronically
irradiated dogs are compared with the responses of dogs given acute bilateral irradiation at 15 R/min, to total doses of ^{60}Co gamma rays
ranging from 275-365 R (Norris et al., 1968).

Dosimetric methods and calculations are outlined in detail elsewhere
(Sinclair, 1963; Williamson et al., 1968; Norris et al., 1968). In
brief, midline daily exposure rates in air were measured with a calibrated ionization chamber coupled with a charge measuring device. Midline
exposures in R, multiplied by individualized fractional absorbed dose
(FAD) values, yielded average absorbed dose estimates in rads for each
irradiated dog. Individualized FAD values were determined mathematically
from a highly correlative linear relationship between the animal's lateral chest dimension (LCD) and the FAD. Approximately 41% of lateral chest
dimensions were estimated (with a maximum 8% error) from chest circumference measurements. The standard LCD/FAD relationship is based on the
experimental dosimetric data reported by Norris et al. (1968), which
accounted for animal size, attenuation and decay factors, as well as
exposure orientation. Linear regression anaysis of the LCD/FAD

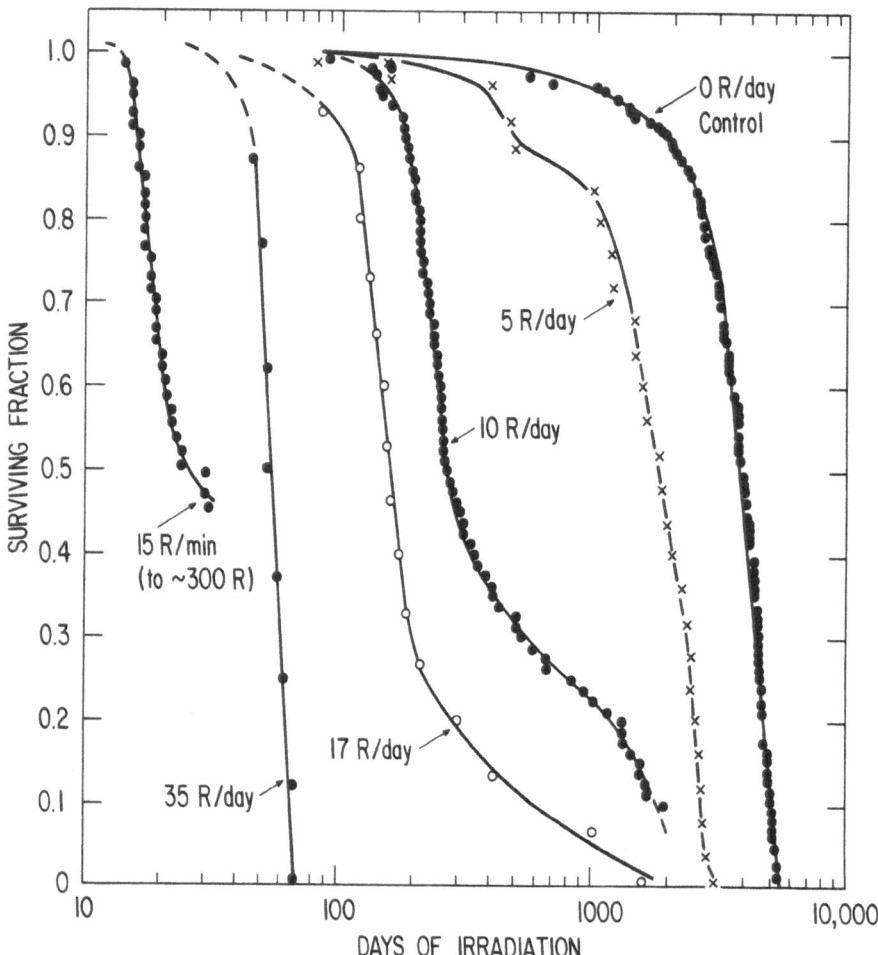

Figure 1. Survival curves based on days of irradiation for groups of beagles exposed to either acute single doses of whole body gamma irradiation (15 R/min; 300 R doses) or continuous low daily doses of whole body gamma irradiation for duration of life (35 to 5 R/22 hr day).

relationship yielded an R^2 value of 0.75 and a slope estimate of
−0.007679 (± 0.000579, S.E.).

Hematology and Pathology

Hemograms were performed by standard methods on each irradiated animal
every 14 days and on each experimental control animal every 28 days
(Tolle et al., 1979a).

When the irradiated animals became acutely ill and moribund, they were
sacrificed by exsanguination while under sodium pentobarbital
anesthesia. Complete necropsies were performed and gross pathological
changes were recorded. Tissue samples were systematically collected and
processed for histological evaluation in order to establish the primary
cause of death.

For the purpose of morphologic and functional analyses of bone marrow
with time and cumulative radiation dose, marrow biopsies and aspirates
were performed at approximately 100-day intervals in selected groups of
animals (10 R/day group; 0 R/day controls). The collected tissue specimens were processed and examined by standard methods (Seed et al., 1977,
1981; Tolle et al., 1979a, 1979b, 1982). The concentrations of hematopoietic progenitors (GM-CFUa) in the biopsied/aspirated marrow samples
were assayed, following a two stage enrichment (glass wool filtration and
ficoll density gradient centrifugation), using modified single-layer
(Marsh et al., 1972) and double-layer (Pike and Robinson, 1970) agar
cloning methods as previously described (Seed et al., 1982). The radiosensitivities of progenitors isolated from both nonirradiated and chronically irradiated animals were analyzed by standard dose response measurements in which marrow cell suspensions (10^6-10^7), enriched in progenitors, were acutely gamma irradiated (25 rads/min) with 0-300 rads.
Degrees of progenitor cell lethality at each dose level were assessed in
terms of the surviving fraction of clonogenically active cells measured
by soft agar cloning (Seed et al., 1982).

RESULTS

Survival Relative to Time and Cumulative Radiation Dose

The survival curves for groups of beagles exposed daily for duration of
life to either 35, 17, 10, or 5 R of whole body ^{60}Co gamma radiation
differ markedly with time (Fig. 1). The estimated median survival times
of irradiated dogs at these daily dose rates are 53, 156, 256, and 1834
days, respectively (Table 1 A-D). These survival times represent fractional life-spans of 1.5, 4.3, 7.1, and 50.8% compared with the extended
median survival time of 3613 days for the nonirradiated colony controls
(i.e., 0 R/day group).

The survival curves based on cumulative dose (Fig. 2), similar to the
curves based on time, are also generally displaced to the right, i.e., to
higher average levels of accumulated radiation dose, as the daily dose
rate of exposure is reduced from very high rates (15 R/min) to very low
rates (5 R/day). From these curves, the LD_{50}'s for continuously delivered whole body gamma irradiation are estimated to be: 1442 rads at a
35 R (27.3 rads) per day exposure rate; 2124 rads at 17 R (13.4 rads) per

142

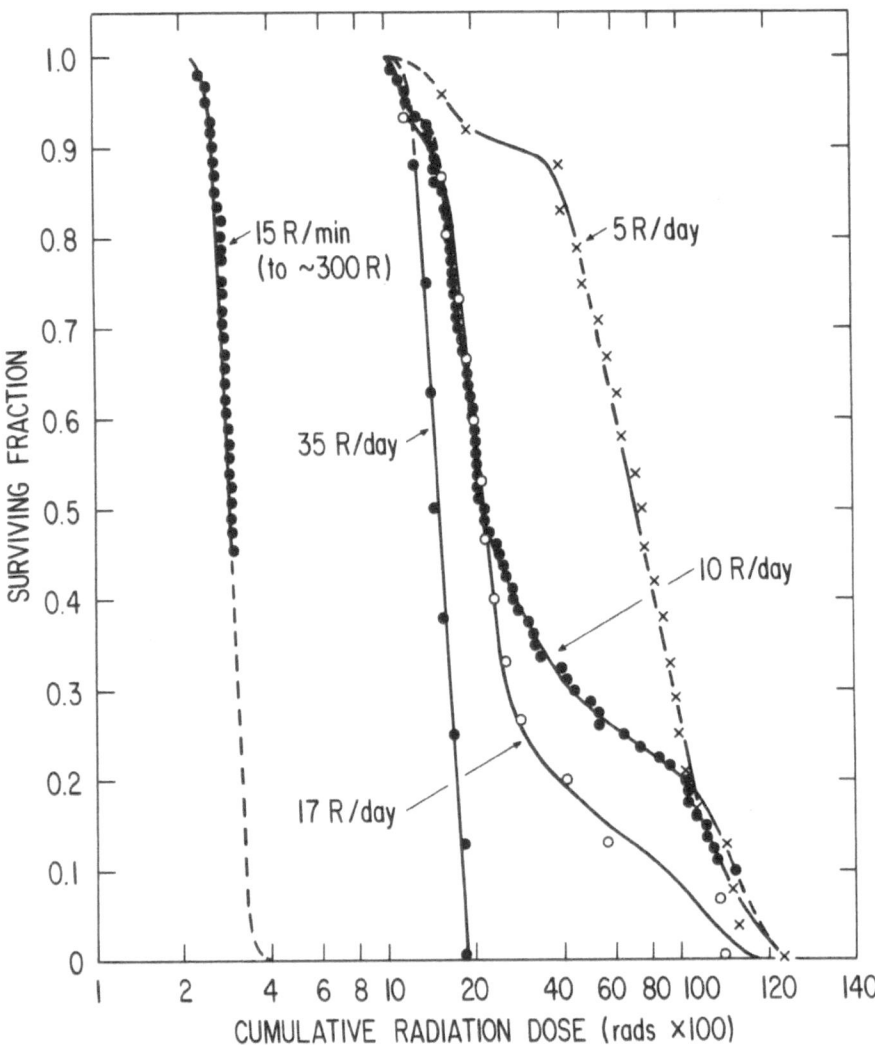

Figure 2. Survival curves based on cumulative dose for groups of beagles exposed to either acute single doses of whole body gamma irradiation (15 R/min; 300 R doses) or continuous low daily doses of whole body gamma irradiation for duration of life (35 to 5 R/22 hr day).

TABLE 1.   Survival and Pathological Responses of Dogs under Chronic Whole Body ^{60}Co Gamma Irradiation: Part A. 35 R/day

Parameters	Group Values [a]	Infect. Disease [b,d]	PRIMARY PATHOLOGIES						
			Hematopoietic Syndromes			H. Diath.	Nonhematopoietic Syndromes		
			Aplasia	MPD	LPD		S. Tumor	Degen. D.	Other
ANIMALS: --									
No.	8	7	1	0	0	0	0	0	0
%	100	87.5	12.5	0	0	0	0	0	0
Relative size[c]	15.7±1.3	15.5±1.3	17.0	--	--	--	--	--	--
RADIATION:									
Daily air dose	35	35	35	--	--	--	--	--	--
Cum. air dose	1991±290	1935±263	2380	--	--	--	--	--	--
Daily absorbed dose	27.3	27.3	27.0	--	--	--	--	--	--
Fract. absorbed dose	0.78±0.01	0.78±0.01	0.77	--	--	--	--	--	--
Cum. absorbed dose	1552±224	1519±209	1831	--	--	--	--	--	--
SURVIVAL:									
Days to death (mean)	57±3	55±8	68	--	--	--	--	--	--
Days to death (median)	53	53	68	--	--	--	--	--	--
LETHALITY:									
Est. LD$_{50}$ (R)	1855	1837	--	--	--	--	--	--	--
Est. LD$_{50}$ (rad)	1442	1426	--	--	--	--	--	--	--

[a] Values listed for animal size, the radiation variables, and survival time are the means ± standard error.
[b] Abbreviations: Infect. disease = infectious diseases (septicemia, pneumonias); MPD = myeloproliferative disorders; LPD = lymphoproliferative disorders (lymphomas, lymphocytic leukemia); H. Diath. = hemorrhagic diathesis; S. Tumor = solid tumor (nonlymphohematopoietic neoplasias); Degen. D. = degenerative diseases.
[c] Relative size values represent the mean (± SE) lateral chest dimension.
[d] At 35 R/day septicemias accounted for 100% of the infectious diseases.

TABLE 1.   Part B.   17 R/day

Parameters	Group[a] Values	Infect.[b,d] Disease	PRIMARY PATHOLOGIES						
			Hematopoietic Syndromes				Nonhematopoietic Syndromes		
			Aplasia	MPD	LPD	H. Diath.	S. Tumor	Degen. D.	Other
ANIMALS:									
No.	15	8	5	2	0	0	0	0	0
%	100	53.3	33.3	13.3	0	0	0	0	0
Relative size[c]	14.3±0.4	14.4±1.6	14.0±0.4	14.5±2.1	--	--	--	--	--
RADIATION:									
Daily air dose	17	17	17	17	--	--	--	--	--
Cum. air dose	5014±1421	2956±673	3254±548	17646±553	--	--	--	--	--
Daily absorbed dose	13.4	13.4	13.4	13.4	--	--	--	--	--
Fract. absorbed dose	0.79±0.01	0.79±0.01	0.79±0.01	0.79±0.02	--	--	--	--	--
Cum. absorbed dose	3961±1120	2338±541	2576±428	13913±149	--	--	--	--	--
SURVIVAL:									
Days to death (mean)	295±84	174±40	191±32	1038±33	--	--	--	--	--
Days to death (median)	156	131	164	1015	--	--	--	--	--
LETHALITY:									
Est. LD_{50} (R)	2661	2227	2780	17255	--	--	--	--	--
Est. LD_{50} (rad)	2124	1753	2211	13808	--	--	--	--	--

[a]Values listed for animal size, the radiation variables, and survival time are the means ± standard error.
[b]Abbreviations: Infect. disease = infectious diseases (septicemia, pneumonias); MPD = myeloproliferative disorders; LPD = lymphoproliferative disorders (lymphomas, lymphocytic leukemia); H. Diath. = hemorrhagic diathesis; S. Tumor = solid tumor (nonlymphohematopoietic neoplasias); Degen. D. = degenerative diseases.
[c]Relative size values represent the mean (± SE) lateral chest dimension.
[d]At 17 R/day septicemias accounted for 100% of the infectious diseases.

TABLE 1. Part C. 10 R/day

Parameters	Group[a] Values	Infect.[b,d] Disease	Hematopoietic Syndromes				Nonhematopoietic Syndromes		
			Aplasia	MPD	LPD	H. Diath.	S. Tumor	Degen. D.	Other
ANIMALS:									
No.	72	8	43	14	1	1	1	2	2
%	100	11.1	59.7	19.4	1.4	1.4	1.4	2.8	2.8
Relative size[c]	13.9±0.2	14.0±0.5	13.7±0.3	13.9±0.5	16.5	13.8	15.0	14.5±2.1	15.4±1.9
RADIATION:									
Daily air dose	10	10	10	10	10	10	10	10	10
Cum. air dose	4744±539	2256±243	1743±308	9006±1327	19660	5280	13320	14895±2298	--
Daily absorbed dose	7.9	7.9	8.0	7.9	7.7	7.9	7.9	7.9	7.8
Fract. absorbed dose	0.79±0.01	0.79±0.01	0.80±0.01	0.79±0.01	0.77	0.79	0.79	0.79±0.01	0.78±0.02
Cum. absorbed dose	3756±425	1786±187	2182±244	7147±1049	15204	4193	10455	1167±2056	4417±2823
SURVIVAL:									
Days to death (mean)	474±54	226±241	274±31	900±133	1966	528	1332	1490±230	568±372
Days to death (median)	256	212	234	669	1966	528	1332	1327	305
LETHALITY:									
Est. LD$_{50}$ (R)	2560	2120	2335	6690	--	--	--	13270	3050
Est. LD$_{50}$ (rad)	2039	1703	1856	5302	--	--	--	10313	2421

[a] Values listed for animal size, the radiation variables, and survival time are the means ± standard error.
[b] Abbreviations: Infect. disease = infectious diseases (septicemia, pneumonias); MPD = myeloproliferative disorders; LPD = lymphoproliferative disorders (lymphomas, lymphocytic leukemia); H. Diath. = hemorrhagic diathesis; S. Tumor = solid tumor (nonlymphohematopoietic neoplasias); Degen. D. = degenerative diseases.
[c] Relative size values represent the mean (± SE) lateral chest dimension.
[d] At 10 R/day septicemias accounted for 87.5% of the infectious processes; pneumonias accounted for 12.5%.

TABLE 1. Part D. 5 R/day

Parameters	Group[a] Values	Infect.[b,d] Disease	Hematopoietic Syndromes				Nonhematopoietic Syndromes		
			Aplasia	MPD	LPD	H. Diath.	S. Tumor	Degen. D.	Other
ANIMALS:									
No.	25	2	2	11	1	0	6	3	0
%	100	8	8	44	4	0	24	12	0
Relative size[c]	14.8±0.2	14.0±1.4	14.7±1.9	15.3±0.9	14	--	14.1±1.3	15.0±0.9	--
RADIATION:									
Daily air dose	5	5	5	5	5	--	5	5	--
Cum. air dose	9150±8201	2185±332	7360±7141	7281±1676	10380	--	13859±1070	12010±838	--
Daily absorbed dose	4.0	4.0	4.0	3.9	--	--	4.0	4.0	--
Fract. absorbed dose	0.79±0.01	0.79±0.02	0.79±0.02	0.78±0.01	0.79	--	0.79±0.01	0.79±0.01	--
Cum. absorbed dose	7199±649	1730±239	5744±5516	5698±1303	8227	--	10977±884	9426±644	--
SURVIVAL:									
Days to death (mean)	1830±164	437±67	1472±1428	1456±335	2076	--	2772±96	2402±119	--
Days to death (median)	1834	390	462	1435	2076	--	2785	2311	--
LETHALITY:									
Est. LD_{50} (R)	9170	1950	2310	7175	--	--	13925	11553	--
Est. LD_{50} (rad)	7161	1561	1843	5605	--	--	10876	9091	--

[a]Values listed for animal size, the radiation variables, and survival time are the means ± standard error.
[b]Abbreviations: Infect. disease = infectious diseases (septicemia, pneumonias); MPD = myeloproliferative disorders; LPD = lymphoproliferative disorders (lymphomas, lymphocytic leukemia); H. Diath. = hemorrhagic diathesis; S. Tumor = solid tumor (nonlymphohematopoietic neoplasias); Degen. D. = degenerative diseases.
[c]Relative size values represent the mean (± SE) lateral chest dimension.
[d]At 5 R/day septicemias accounted for 100% of the infectious diseases.

day; 2039 rads at 10 R (7.9 rads) per day; and 7161 rads at 5 R (4.0 rads) per day (Table 1 A-D).

In contrast to the clearly separate, time-dependent survival responses (Fig. 1), the survival responses based on cumulative dose (individualized rad dose) at 17 and 10 R/day are nearly identical in the initial, linear portion of the curves below the 90% survival level. Below 50% survival there are obvious transitions to lower lethality rates. Similar, but less abrupt transitions also occur in the time-dependent survival curves at these intermediate dose rates (Fig. 1). These lethality rate transitions occur following cumulative doses of ~ 2500 rads at the 25% and 40% survival levels at 17 R/day and 10 R/day, respectively (Figs. 1 and 2).

Survival Times, Pathologies, and Estimated LD_{50}'s of Subgroups

Transitions in rates of lethality at the intermediate dose rates reflect and highlight the inherent heterogeneity of the population relative to the radiosensitivity and the pathological tendencies of its individuals. As indicated in Table 1 A-E, the overall spectrum of developing primary pathologies (as major contributors to the lethality response patterns) shifts from a predominance of the early arising lymphohematopoietic syndromes (i.e., septicemias and aplastic anemias) at the higher, functionally ablative, radiation dose rates to a predominance of the late arising hematopoietic and nonhematopoietic neoplasias and degenerative disorders at the lower, less lymphohematopoietically ablative dose rates.

The pathological responses of the nonirradiated control animals (Table 1 E) illustrate the spectrum and incidences of pathologies at background levels of exposure. The very late developing nonhematopoietic syndromes, principally solid tumors, are largely responsible for the overall lethality. The early arising acute lymphohematopoietic syndromes, characteristic responses under high dose rate exposure, do not contribute to the lethality. Infectious diseases contribute minimally, and are mainly in the form of late occurring pneumonias rather than the early occurring radiation-associated septicemias. Late arising myeloproliferative disorders do not occur. The lymphoproliferative syndromes (i.e., lymphomas and lymphocytic leukemias) occur in the controls at slightly elevated incidences (7.3%) when compared with the 4.0% and 1.4% incidences at the 5 and 10 R/day dose rate levels.

The pathological spectrum at the intermediate dose rate of 10 R/day, in contrast to either the high or low dose rate extremes, encompasses in sizable numbers both early and late arising hematopoietic syndromes, as well as the nonhematopoietic syndromes (Table 1 C). This broad pathological spectrum is largely responsible for the previously noted time and cumulative dose-dependent transitions in the lethality rate (Figs. 1 and 2). The initially steep sloped lethality curve is mainly due to the early development of lethal aplasias, whereas the late developing myeloproliferative disorders (mainly granulocytic leukemia) appear to be the principal reason for the noted transition to the lower time and cumulative dose-dependent rate of lethality.

These markedly different pathological and survival responses to different exposure rates of continuous irradiation, within a relatively homogeneous group of purebred beagles maintained under standard conditions, indicate

TABLE 1. Part E. Nonirradiated Controls

Parameters	Group[a] Values	Infect.[b,d] Disease	PRIMARY PATHOLOGIES Hematopoietic Syndromes				Nonhematopoietic Syndromes		
			Aplasia	MPD	LPD	H. Diath.	S. Tumor	Degen. D.	Other
ANIMALS:									
No.	96	11	0	0	7	0	42	11	25
%	100	11.5	0	0	7.3	0	43.8	11.5	26.0
Relative size[c]	--	--	--	--	--	--	--	--	--
RADIATION:									
Daily air dose	0	0	0	0	0	0	0	0	0
Cum. air dose	--	--	--	--	--	--	--	--	--
Daily absorbed dose	--	--	--	--	--	--	--	--	--
Fract. absorbed dose	--	--	--	--	--	--	--	--	--
Cum. absorbed dose	--	--	--	--	--	--	--	--	--
SURVIVAL[e]:									
Days to death (mean)	3377±139	2751±385	--	--	3767±538	--	3960±142	3247±513	2646±312
Days to death (median)	3613 (3700)	2617	--	--	4308	--	4094	2822	2790
LETHALITY:									
Est. LD$_{50}$ (R)	NA	NA	--	--	--	--	NA	NA	NA
Est. LD$_{50}$ (rad)	NA	NA	--	--	--	--	NA	NA	NA

[a]Values listed for animal size, the radiation variables, and survival time are the means ± standard error.
[b]Abbreviations: Infect. disease = infectious diseases (septicemia, pneumonias); MPD = myeloproliferative disorders; LPD = lymphoproliferative disorders (lymphomas, lymphocytic leukemia); H. Diath. = hemorrhagic diathesis; S. Tumor = solid tumor (nonlymphohematopoietic neoplasias); Degen. D. = degenerative diseases.
[c]Relative size values represent the mean (± SE) lateral chest dimension.
[d]At 0 R/day septicemias accounted for 9% of the infectious disease cases, pneumonias 91%.
[e]The mean/median survival times during the experiment (experimental survival + 400 days = chronological survival time) are based on 96 decedents within the control group of 153 dogs, of which 57 are still alive. The median value is (in parentheses) based on the total group of 153 animals; the survival times of the 57 living dogs are factored in.

that there may be several subgroups within the population with varying radiation sensitivities and pathological predispositions. Based on this subgroup concept, we have estimated LD_{50}'s for each of the major pathological categories. For the most part, these pathology-specific LD_{50} values appear reasonably close among the various dose rates of exposure. The differences are less than would be expected if the development of the hematopoietic syndromes was totally dose-rate dependent. The ranges of the estimated LD_{50}'s for the following subgroups are (a) infectious diseases, 1426-1753 rads at 35-10 R/day; (b) aplastic anemia, 1856-2211 rads at 17 and 10 R/day; (c) myeloproliferative diseases (MPD), 5302-5605 rads at 10 and 5 R/day (13808 rads for the two dogs at 17 R/day); (d) nonhematopoietic tumors, 10876 rads at 5 R/day; and (e) degenerative diseases, 9091 rads at 5 R/day.

Hematologic Responses of the Major Subgroups

Examination of the peripheral blood responses of the aplasia subgroup (Fig. 3 A-F) and the myeloproliferative subgroup (Fig. 4 A-F), relative to the nonirradiated controls (Fig. 5 A-F) revealed a major developmental difference in the pathological progression of these two end points. Both subgroups initially responded to the hemotoxic effects of continuous whole body gamma irradiation by rapid and progressive decline in circulating levels of platelets and granulocytes (Figs. 3 B,E and 4 B,E). However, once the nadir of the platelet or granulocyte response was reached, at approximately 150-200 days, the MPD subgroup initiated a reparative hematopoietic process, as evidenced by a gradual, partial restoration of circulating blood levels of platelets, leukocytes (total granulocyte and immature neutrophils), and, to a limited extent, erythrocytes (Fig. 3 A-F). The aplasia subgroup, in contrast, failed to initiate this reparative phase, as evidenced by the maintenance of extremely low blood cell levels, resulting in the development of acute, terminal pancytopenic conditions (Fig. 4 A-F).

The bone marrow responses to the continuous irradiation (i.e., changing pool sizes of granulocyte/monocyte progenitors) compared with peripheral blood changes had similar patterns in the two subgroups (Fig. 6). In both subgroups, GM-progenitor marrow compartments were progressively depleted to less than 10% of their preirradiation sizes over the first 100 days of exposure (representing cumulative doses of 790-800 rads). In contrast to the continued depletion and eventual sterilization of this vital progenitor compartment within the aplasia subgroup, the long surviving MPD subgroup reversed the potentially lethal, acutely progressive myelosuppressive response with the initiation of a reparative process, evidenced by the slow, gradual increased size of the GM-progenitor marrow compartment.

The expansion of the GM-progenitor marrow compartment in the face of continued daily irradiation suggests that the initially radiosensitive marrow progenitors acquired increased radioresistance at or about the time the repair process was initiated. This suggestion of acquired radioresistance at the progenitor cell level is supported by direct in vitro testing of the radiosensitivity of isolated GM-progenitors from the aplasia and MPD subgroups (Seed et al., 1982). The radioresistance of postrecovery GM-progenitors isolated from MPD subgroups was markedly increased in contrast to the relatively low radioresistance of

150

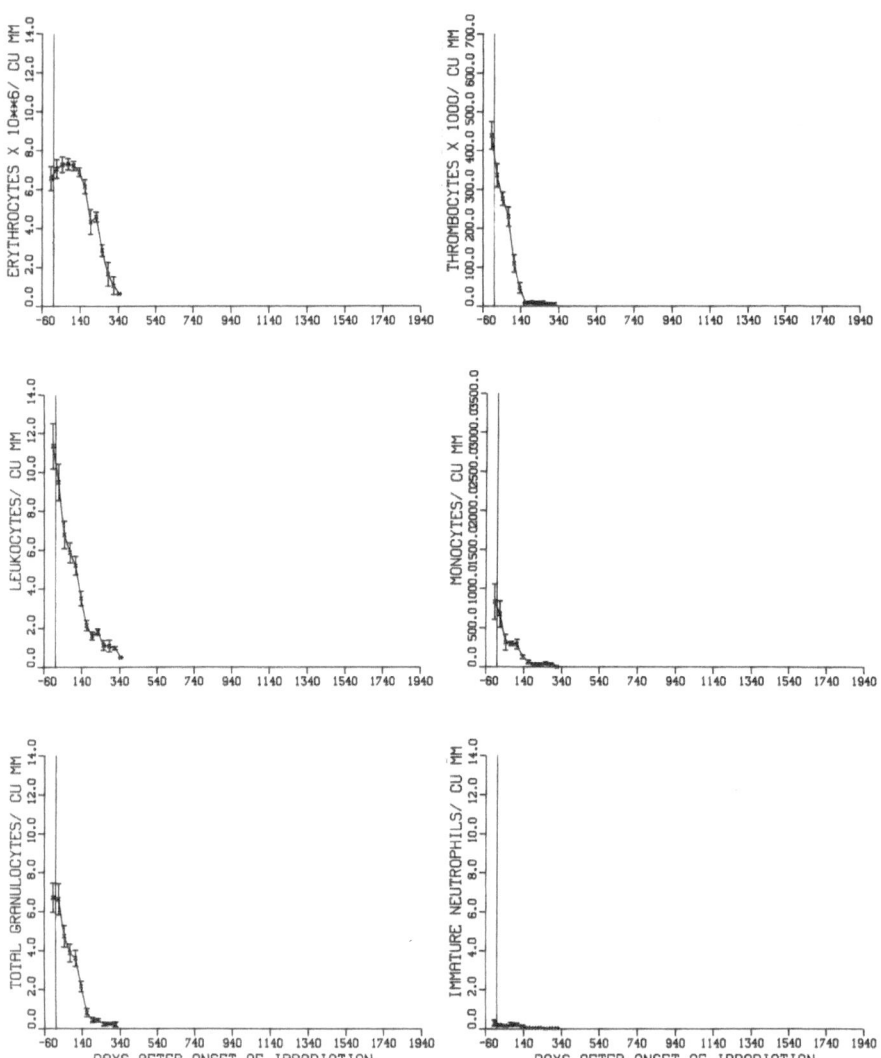

Figure 3. Peripheral blood responses of continuously irradiated (10 R/day) beagles with developing aplastic anemia. A, erythrocytes; B, blood platelets or thrombocytes; C, total leukocytes; D, monocytes; E, total granulocytes; and F, immature neutrophils (granulocytes). Note the survival course and the progressive decline in blood cell levels and the absence of hematopoietic recovery.

MYELOPROLIFERATIVE SUBGROUP

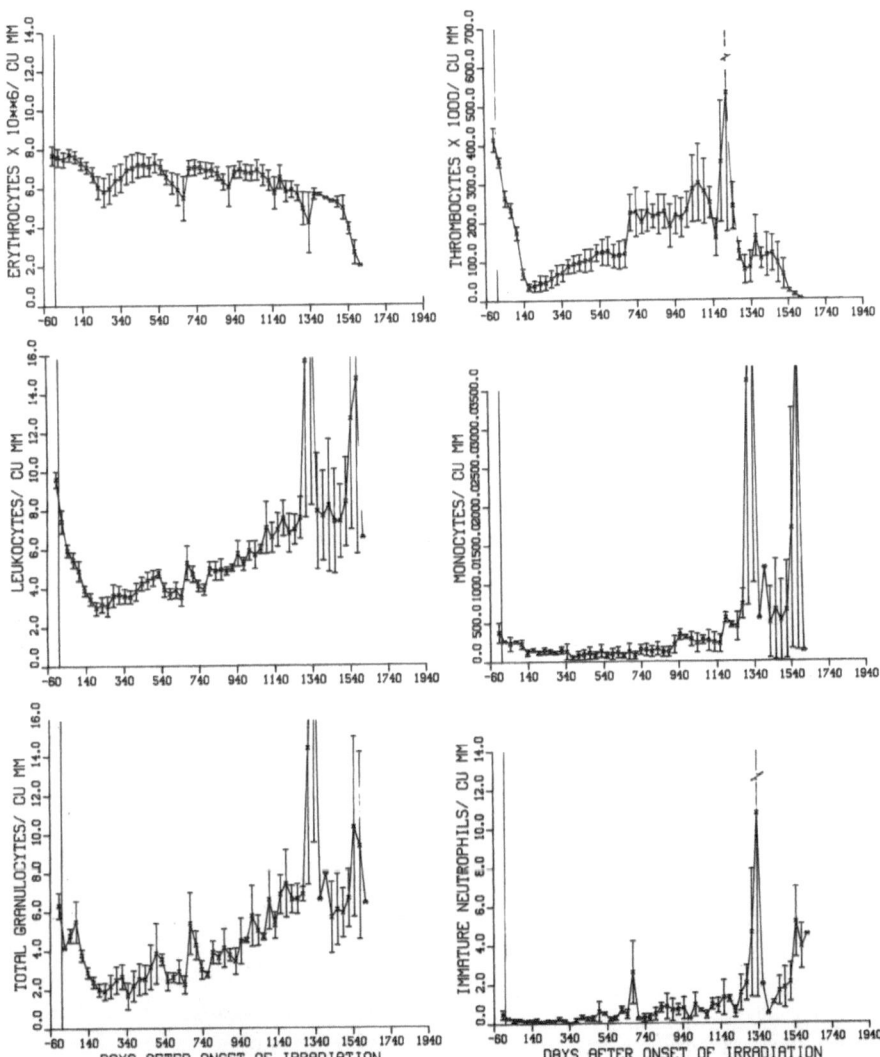

Figure 4. Peripheral blood responses of continuously irradiated (10 R/day) beagles with developing myeloproliferative disorders, principally myelogenous leukemia. The cell type under assessment is marked on the Y-axis. In contrast to the aplasia subgroup, the myeloproliferative disease subgroup exhibits prolonged survival and pronounced recovery phaes at approximately 150-250 days.

152

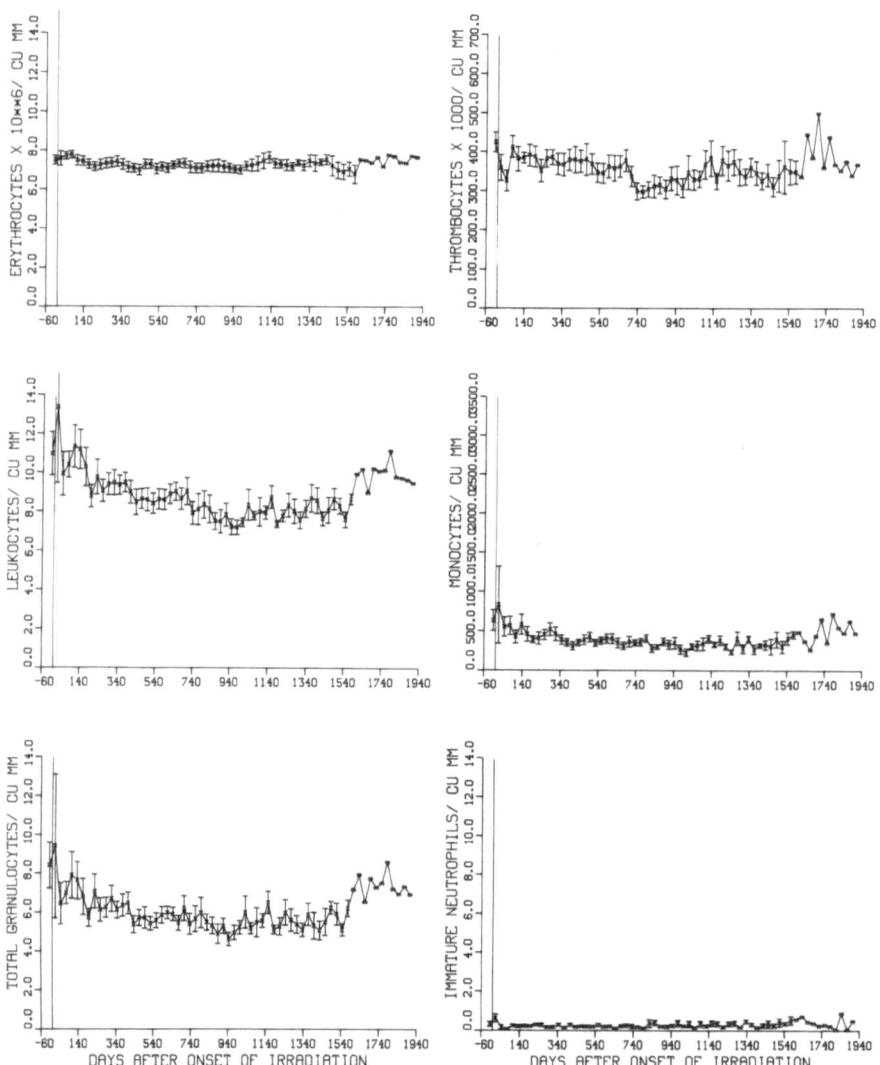

Figure 5. Peripheral blood values of nonirradiated control dogs. Cell type under assessment is marked on the Y-axis.

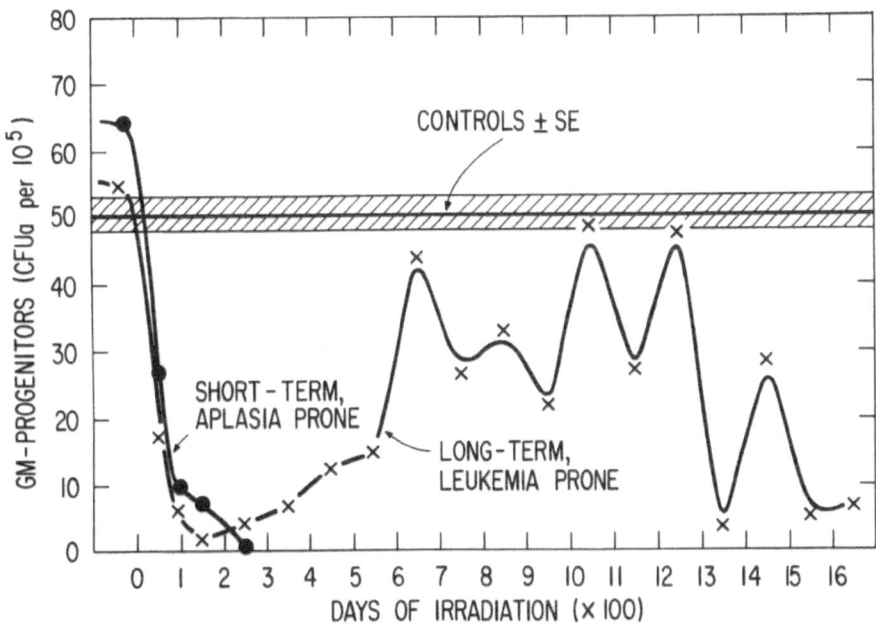

Figure 6. Sequential change with time of irradiation in bone marrow (iliac crest) concentrations of granulocyte/monocyte progenitors in dogs with progressing aplastic anemia (●) or leukemia (X) (part of the myeloproliferative disease complex). Note different responses of the two subgroups relative to recovery of marrow progenitor levels. (Redrawn from Seed et al., 1982.)

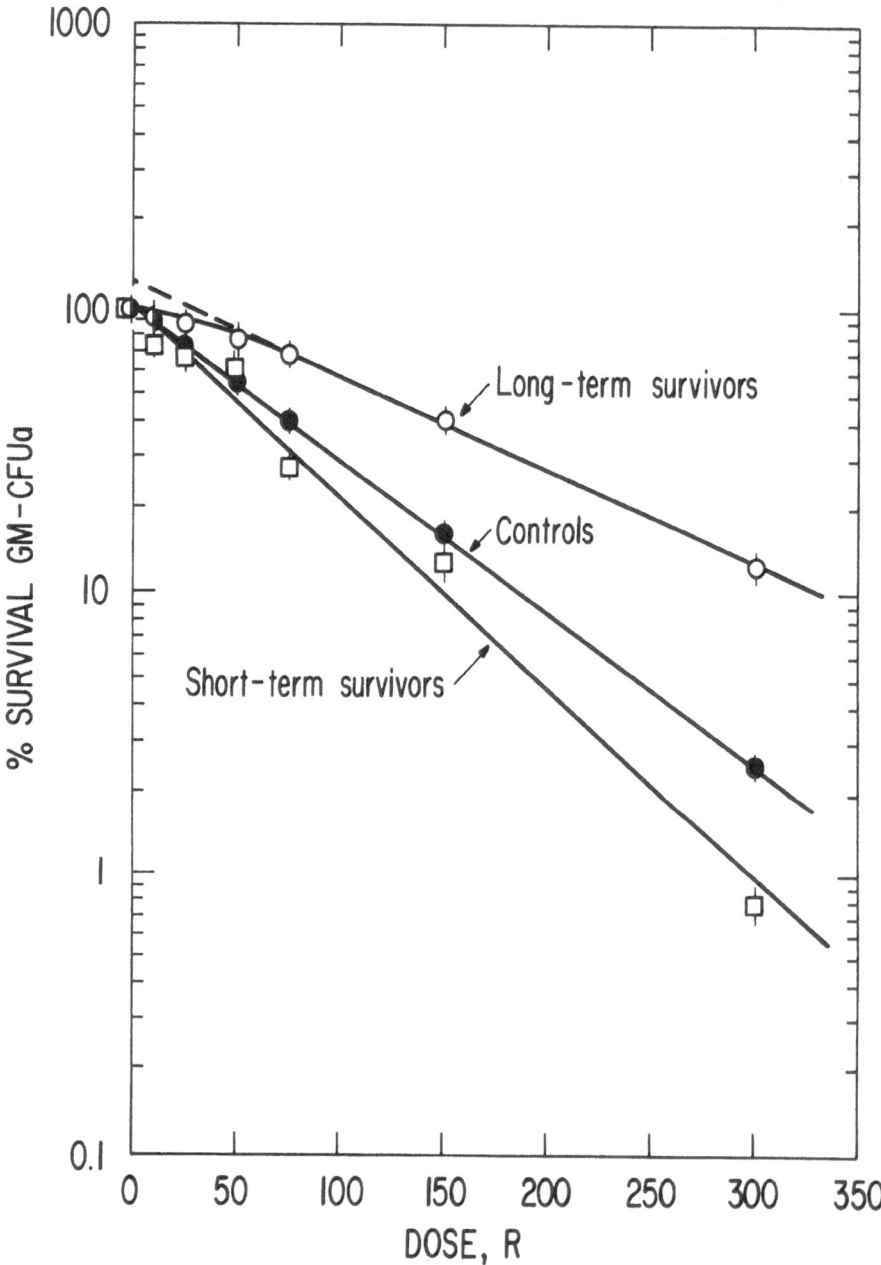

Figure 7. Radiosensitivity of GM-progenitors isolated from aplasia-prone, short-term survivors (□), myeloproliferative disease-prone, long-term survivors (○), or from nonirradiated control animals (●). Note the marked increased radioresistance of progenitors of the MPD-prone dogs following the period of hematopoeitic recovery. (From Seed et al., 1982.)

GM-progenitors from either the aplasia subgroup or from nonirradiated control dogs (Fig. 7).

DISCUSSION

Nearly three decades ago, Sacher (1955) and Mole (1957) recognized the relationships among the daily rate of ionizing radiation exposure, the extent of life shortening, and the change in the effective per unit dose with protraction of exposure. Subsequent analyses by Grahn and Sacher (Grahn and Sacher, 1968; Sacher et al., 1978) characterized a specific radiation parameter that defined the degree of life shortening for a given species under various exposure regimens. This parameter (K), defined by the regression coefficient of the mean aftersurvival/dose rate relationship, was suggested to be "virtually a species constant," and not altered by minor strain differences within a given species (Grahn and Sacher, 1968). From this work, Sacher et al. (1978) developed a generic, radiation-specific lethality rate/dose rate relationship: i.e., lethality rates shift from dose rate independence at very low daily exposure rates, to dose rate dependence at intermediate exposure rates, and back to dose rate independence at very high exposure rates. The specific dose rates (break points) at which these transitions occur appear to be characteristic of the irradiated species.

In agreement with Grahn and Sacher's analyses, we have observed marked changes in the lethality rates of continuously irradiated beagles over a 35-5 R/day range of exposure rates. As predicted, the calculated radiation-specific lethality rates (based on mean aftersurvival times (Sacher et al., 1978) increased linearly (log/log plot) in a dose rate dependent fashion. However, our lethality rate calculations based on cumulative absorbed dose are not nearly as linear, due to the similar lethality rates at the intermediate exposure rates of 17 R and 10 R/day.

The major transitions in lethality rates, from dose rate dependency, clearly involve the lymphohematopoietic system and its response to accumulated radiation-induced injury. Transitions at high dose rates occur as the result of the reaching and exceeding of maximum sterilizing rates of vital proliferative lymphohematopoietic tissue. Transitions at very low dose rates are thought to be the consequence of the sparing of lymphohematopoietic function, which enables a time-dependent expression of late arising, nonhematopoietic syndromes. The latter concept is supported in this study by the noted increased contribution of the nonhematopoietic syndromes, relative to the lymphohematopoietic disorders, to the overall lethality response at very low (5 R/day) or background levels (zero R/day) of exposure.

The lethality rate transitions occur over a "range" of exposure rates (i.e., inter-dose rate transitions). We have observed similar lethality rate transitions within groups of animals exposed at the "same" daily rate (i.e., intra-dose rate transitions). Such intra-dose rate transitions in lethality rate, in contrast to the inter-dose rate transitions, appear to arise as a result of the shift in incidence of specific hematopathologies; the initially high rate of lethality observed at the 17 and 10 R/day levels is due to early developing aplastic anemias, whereas the secondary, lower rate of lethality is largely the result of the late developing myeloproliferative disorders. The latter association suggests the presence of distinct subgroups within the population, characterized by differences in radiosensitivity and pathological tendencies.

In terms of hematopoietic function, the radiosensitive, aplasia-prone subgroup and the radioresistant, MPD-prone subgroup are distinguished by the repair capacity of hematopoietic tissue under continuous irradiation (Seed et al., 1977, 1978, 1981, 1982). It is this single capacity that appears to mediate the previously noted lethality rate transitions (i.e., intra-dose rate transitions) and, ultimately, the shift from the nonneoplastic to neoplastic hematopathologies.

The cellular basis of this repair capacity appears to involve, in part, an acquisition of radioresistance by vital hematopoietic progenitors (Seed et al., 1982, 1983). In vitro correlates of such acquired radioresistance by hematopoietic cells under chronic irradiation are well documented (Lamerton and Courtenay, 1968; Courtenay, 1969; Gregg et al., 1979) and support the concept of acquired radioresistance by early hematopoietic progenitors as a mediator of hematopoietic repair, and in turn accommodation under chronic irradiation in vivo. This concept does not discount the possibility that other mechanisms are operative: namely, enhanced progenitor cell cycling (Gidali et al., 1979; Wu and Lajtha, 1975), reduced cell cycle times of proliferative elements (Lord, 1964), broadening of the proliferative zones (Lamerton, 1966), and increased transit marrow times of maturing cells (Lamerton et al., 1968).

Regardless of the cellular mechanism, the repair process occurs and is largely, if not totally, responsible for the transition from the nonneoplastic to neoplastic hematopathologies seen under continuous gamma irradiation at intermediate dose rate levels (17 and 10 R/day).

From a biological viewpoint, it is ironic that the very process that spares the chronically irradiated animal from one type of hematopoietic disease (e.g., aplastic anemia) serves to foster a second type (e.g., granulocytic leukemia). Indeed, the "price paid" by the animal for being "rescued" from ablative hematopoietic syndromes, via the acquisition of repair functions, is not inexpensive.

ACKNOWLEDGMENTS

The authors gratefuly acknowledge the assistance of Mrs. Laverne Bell and Mrs. Carol Fox for computer services and data management, Mr. William Keenan for clinical services, Dr. Marcia Rosenthal for her editorial assistance, and Ms. Lynn Purdy for secretarial help and assistance in preparation of the manuscript. We also thank the Argonne Animal Care Specialists for their daily care of the research animals and maintenance of facilities accredited by the American Association for Accreditation of Laboratory Animal Care. Work supported by U.S. Department of Energy under contract No. W-31-109-ENG-38 and by the National Cancer Institute, U.S. Department of Health and Human Services under agreement Y01-CO-00-320.

REFERENCES

Blackett, N.M. Erythropoiesis in the rat under continuous gamma irradiation. Brit. J. Haemat. 13: 915-33 (1967).

Brown, D.G., Cragle, R.G. Some observations of dose-rate effect of radiation on burros, swine, and cattle. In: Dose Rate in Radiation Biology, CONF-680410, pp. 5.1-5.16, US Atomic Energy Commission, Oak Ridge, TN (1968).

Bustad, L.K., Gates, N.M., Ross, A., Carlson, L.D. Effects of prolonged low-level irradiation of mice. Radiat. Res. 25: 318-330 (1965).

Courtenay, V.D. Radioresistant mutants of L5178Y cells. Radiat. Res. 38: 186-203 (1969).

Fritz, T.E., Norris, W.P., Tolle, D.V., Seed, T.M., Poole, C.M., Lombard, L.S., and Doyle, D.E. Relationship of dose rate and total dose to responses of continuously irradiated beagles. In: Late Biological Effects of Ionizing Radiation, vol. 2, pp. 71-82, IAEA-SM-224/206, International Atomic Energy Agency, Vienna (1978).

Fritz, T.E., Tolle, D.V., Doyle, D.E., Seed, T.M., Cullen, S.M. Hematologic responses of beagles exposed continuosuly to low doses of ^{60}Co gamma-radiation. In: Experimental Hematology Today 1982, S.J. Baum, G.D. Ledney, S.T. Thierfelder, (eds.) pp. 229-240, S. Karger, Basel (1982).

Gidali, J., Bojtor, I., Feher, I. Kinetic basis for compensated hemopoiesis during continuous irradiation with low doses. Radiat. Res. 77: 285-291 (1979).

Grahn, D., Sacher, G.A. Fractination and protraction factors and the late effects of radiation in small mammals. In: Dose Rate in Mammalian Radiation Biology, CONF-680410, pp. 2.1-2.7, US Atomic Energy Commission, Oak Ridge, TN (1968).

Gregg, E.C., Yau, T.M., Kin, S.C. Effect of low dose rate radiation on cell growth kinetics. Biophys. J. 28: 81-91 (1979).

Kalina, I., Praslicka, M. Changes in hemopoiesis and survival of mice exposed to long-term radiation. Radiobiologiya 17: 849-854 (1977).

Lamerton, L.F., Pontifex, A.H., Blackett, N.M., Adams, K. Effects of protracted irradiation on the blood-forming organs of the rat: I. Continuous exposure. Brit. J. Radiol. 33: 287-301 (1960).

Lamerton, L.F. Cell proliferation under continuous irradation. Radiat. Res. 27: 119-138 (1966).

Lamerton, L.V., Courtenay, V.D. The steady state under continuous irradiation. In: Dose Rate in Mammalian Radiation Biology, CONF-680410, pp. 3.2-3.12, US Atomic Energy Commission, Oak Ridge, TN (1968).

Lord, B.I. The effects of continuous irradiation on cell proliferation in rat bone marrow. Brit. J. Haemat. 10: 496-507 (1964).

Lord, B.I. Haemopoietic changes in the rat during growth and during continuous gamma irradiation of the adult animal. Brit. J. Haemat. 11: 525-536 (1965).

Marsh, J., Levitt, M., Katzenstein, A. The growth of leukocyte colonies in vitro from dog bone marrow. J. Lab. Clin. Med. 79: 1041-1050 (1972).

Mole, R.H. Quantitative observations on recovery from whole body irradiation in mice. II. Recovery during and after daily irradiation. Brit. J. Radiol. 30: 40-46 (1957).

Norris, W.P., Fritz, T.E., Rehfeld, C.E., and Poole, C.M. The response of the beagle dog to cobalt-60 gamma radiation: Determination of the LD50(30) and description of associated changes. Radiat. Res. 35: 681-708 (1968).

Norris, W.P., Fritz T.E. Interactions of total dose and dose rate in determining tissue responses to ionizing radiations. In: Radiobiology of Plutonium, B.J. Stover and W.S.S. Jee, (eds) pp. 243-260, J. W. Press, University of Utah, Salt Lake City (1972).

Page, N.P., Ainsworth, E.J., Leong, G.F. The relationship of exposure rate and exposure and exposure time to radiation injury in sheep. Radiat. Res. 33: 94-106 (1968).

Pike, B.L., Robinson, W.A. Human bone marrow colony growth in agargel. J. hysiol. 76: 77-84 (1970).

Pontifex, A.H., Lamerton, L.F. Effects of protracted irradiation on the blood-forming organs of the rat. II. Divided doses. Brit. J. Radiol. 396: 736-747 (1960).

Sacher, G.A. A comparative analysis of radiation lethality in mammals exposed at constant average intensity for the duration of life. J. Natl. Canc. Inst. 15: 1125-1144 (1955).

Sacher, G.A., Tyler, S.A., Trucco, E. The quadratic Low-LET dose-effect relation for life shortening in mammals: Implications for the assessment of the low-dose hazard to human populations. In: Late Biological Effects of Ionizing Radiation, vol. II, IAEA-SM-224/408, pp. 359-375, International Atomic Energy Agency, Vienna (1978).

Seed, T.M., Tolle, D.V., Fritz, T.E., Devine, R.L., Poole, C.M., Norris, W.P. Irradiation-induced erythroleukemia and myelogenous leukemia in the beagle dog: Hematology and ultrastructure. Blood 50: 1061-1079 (1977).

Seed, T.M., Tolle, D.V., Fritz, T.E., Cullen, S.M., Kaspar, L.V., Poole, C.M. Haemopathological consequences of protracted gamma irradiation in the beagle. Preclinical phases of leukemia induction. In: Late Biological Effects of Ionizing Radiation, vol. 1, IAEA-SM-224/308, pp. 531-545, International Atomic Energy Agency, Vienna (1978).

Seed, T.M., Cullen, S.M., Kaspar, L.V., Tolle, D.V., Fritz, T.E. Hemopathologic consequences of protracted gamma irradiation: Alteration in granulocyte reserves and granulocyte mobilization. Blood 56: 42-51 (1980).

Seed, T.M., Chubb, G.T., Tolle, D.V. Sequential changes in bone marrow architecture during continuous low dose gamma irradiation. Scan. Elect. Microsc. 1981: 61-72 (1981).

Seed, T.M., Kaspar, L.V., Tolle, D.V., Fritz, T.E. Hemopathologic predisposition and survival time under continuous gamma irradiation: Responses mediated by altered radiosensitivity and hemopoietic progenitors. Exp. Hematol. 10 (suppl. 12): 232-248 (1982).

Seed, T.M., Kaspar, L.V., Tolle, D.V., Fritz, T.E. Acquired radioresistance of hematopoietic progenitors under continuous low daily dose gamma irradiation. Exp. Hematol. (1983, in press).

Sinclair, W.K. Absorbed dose in biological specimens irradiated externally with cobalt-60 gamma radiation. Radiat. Res. 20: 288-297 (1963).

Tolle, D.V., Seed, T.M., Fritz, T.E., Norris, W.P. Irradiation-induced canine leukemia: A proposed new model. Incidence and hematopathology. In: Experimental Hematology Today 1979, S.J. Baum, G.D. Ledney, (eds) pp. 247-256, Springer-Verlag, New York (1979a).

Tolle, D.V., Seed, T.M., Fritz, T.E., Lombard, L.S., Poole, C.M., Norris, W.P. Acute monocytic leukemia in an irradiated beagle. Vet. Pathol. 16: 243-254 (1979b).

Tolle, D.V., Fritz, T.E., Seed, T.M., Cullen, S.M., Lombard, L.S., Poole, C.M. Leukemia induction in beagles exposed continuously to ^{60}Co γ-irradiation: Hematopathology. In: Experimental Hematology Today 1982, S.J. Baum, G.D. Ledney, S. Thierfelder, (eds) pp. 241-249, S. Karger, Basel (1982).

Twentyman, P.R., Blackett, N.M. Red cell production in the continuously irradiated mouse. Brit. J. Radiol. 43: 898-902 (1970).

Williamson, F.S., Hubbard, L.B., Jordan, D.L. The responses of beagle dogs to protracted exposure to ^{60}Co gamma rays at 5-35 R/day. 1. Dosimetry. In: Annual Report 1968, Biological and Medical Research Division, ANL-7535, pp. 153-156, Argonne National Laboratory, Argonne, Illinois (1968).

Wu, C.T., Lajtha, L.G. Haemopoietic stem-cell kinetics during continuous irradiation. Int. J. Radiat. Biol. 27: 41-50 (1975).

HAEMATOPOIETIC SYNDROME IN PIGS

G. Lemaire and J. Maas

Groupe Mixte de Recherche, CEA-DRET,
Fontenay-aux-Roses, France

Introduction

In preliminary studies carried out to determine the RBE of fission neutrons versus that of cobalt 60 gamma radiation the criterion retained was the mean lethal dose within 30 days (LD 50/30) in piglets.

In order to show roughly that the RBE of fission neutrons was greater than 1 for this criterion in large mammals in spite of differences found in the literature (1-12), the method of exposure was unilateral and the mid-line tissue dose was chosen as reference dose. In mixed neutron-gamma fluences, unilateral exposure is ipso facto heterogeneous according to the definitions formulated by the ICRU (13).

These reasons were the basis of the choice of the experimental conditions and the study of the haematopoietic syndrome, responsible for mortality within thirty days following the acute irradiation of the organism. Only clinical symptoms shown by the animals were analysed, as well as blood cell concentrations and the macroscopic lesions found during autopsy.

Materials and Methods

Animals

These were female piglets, the first generation of a Large White and Land Race cross, aged about 2 months and weighing between 16 and 20 kg. A week before their exposure the animals were put in an animal-laboratory unit (IFFA-CREDO) set up near the radiation sources. They stayed there in individual cages at a temperature of 20 ± 1° C and in light conditions which provided alternating daylight and darkness every 12 hours. Food, in the form of granules, was given morning and evening fifteen minutes before the drinking water.

A tranquillizing agent, Azaperone (Stresnil, N.D.), was administered subcutaneously before the piglet was put in a hammock. The animal was then taken to the exposure chamber and placed on a mobile carrier.

Exposure was done individually in the pure gamma fluence and four to six animals at a time in the mixed fluence. In the latter case their sagittal plan was on a concentric circle at 3 to 4 m from the axis of the reactor vessel, the left flank in a proximal position, the centre of the body at 1.2 m from the ground.

Twelve piglets were irradiated. A thirteenth, sham-irradiated, served as control. Before and after exposure, the piglets were examined for clinical signs (morning and evening) and haematological changes (at regular intervals).

162

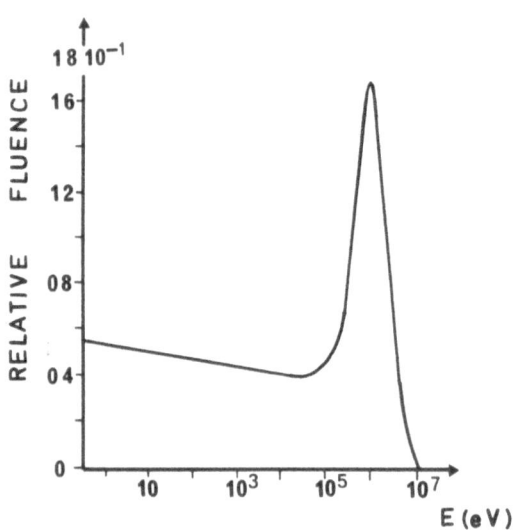

Figure 1: Energy spectrum of neutrons from the bare Silène reactor.

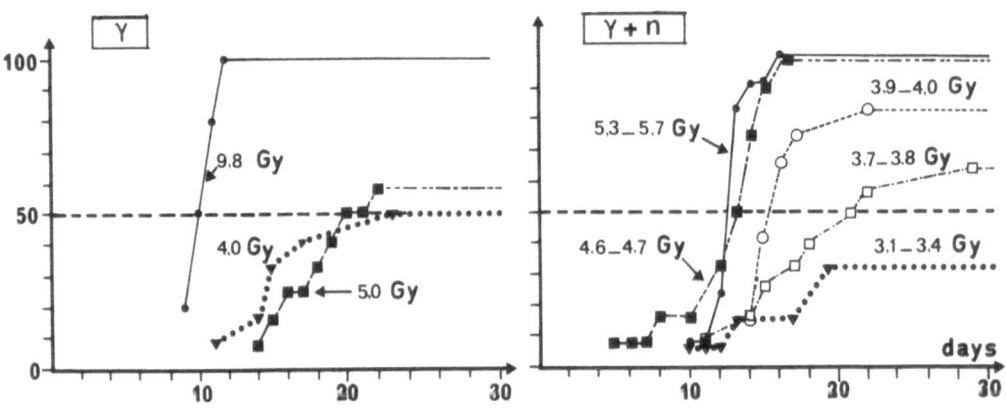

Figure 2: Cumulative mortality in pigs unilaterally irradiated with gamma rays and mixed neutron-gamma radiation. The doses are expressed as midline tissue dose free-in-air.

Blood samples were taken from the auricular vein. Heparin pipettes of 40 µl were filled by capillarity with blood flowing freely from the needle, which was 0.6 mm in diameter. The contents of each pipette was immediately transferred into the Isoton II of Coultronics (20 ml for the red or white cell counts, 2 ml for the platelet count). Smears were also made to establish the leukocyte differential count after colouring by the May Grünwald stain, and to determine the percentage of reticulocytes after colouring by cresyl blue. Each sampling was done twice.

Gamma irradiations

A cobalt 60 irradiator was used which delivered in the tissues an absorbed dose rate varying between 0.1 and 0.08 Gy per min at 1.4 m. The field defined by the collimator is adequate for the dose delivered to the whole animal to be homogeneous to more than 6% compared with the dose delivered only in the axis of the source. Before each exposure, the pig, at 1.4 m from the source, was placed so that the axis of the beam passed through the central point of the animal (located half-way between the occipital ridge and the base of the tail).

Dosimetry of the gamma fluence was carried out with the aid of a tissue equivalent ionization chamber of 5 ml volume coupled with a Novelec electrometer. The central point of the chamber is placed where the centre of the animal would be if it were in the exposure position. The chamber had been previously calibrated in a Cobalt 60 gamma beam at the Etablissement Technique Central de l'Armement (ARCUEIL), which also carried out the metrology of the exposure cell. The experimentally measured values of the gamma-ray absorbed dose always corresponded to less than 3% with those deduced by decay (half-life 5.27 years) from the dose output measured previously.

Mixed neutron-gamma irradiations

The Silène reactor at the Section d'Etudes Expérimentales de Sûreté Nucléaire et Criticité, Institut de Protection et Sûreté Nucléaire, VALDUC, was used. In the method of procedure (flash) an extremely energetic and short power reaction (lasting 10^{-3} s) is provoked by extracting a rod absorbing the neutrons of the uranyl nitrate solution. This solution fills the reactor vessel to a supercritical level predetermined according to the excess of reactivity required by the experiment. The radiation field in a configuration without shield is characterized by a ratio of gamma-neutron dose around 1.2. The isotropy of the flux of particles was verified and, as the reactor core is in a very large room, the diffused radiation was negligible compared with the direct radiation. The neutron spectrum without shield is shown in Figure 1.

Dosimetry of the mixed neutron-gamma fluence as described elsewhere (14) was carried out by the Laboratoire de Dosimetrie Sanitaire, Département de Protection at Fontenay-aux-Roses. It was completed by a detailed study of the dose absorbed inside a pig's carcass of the same volume, from the practical point of view (implantation in different areas, especially medullary, of diodes only sensitive to neutrons which energy is greater than 200 keV and of thermoluminescent dosimeters) and from the theoretical point of view (Monte-Carlo calculations from the spectrum of emitted neutrons). The physical dosimetry was completed by measurement of phosphorus 32 induced by the (n, p) reaction with the sulphur 32 present in the hair (bristles).

Results

The doses (mid-line tissue dose) tested up to now are summarized in Table I.

Table I

LD 50/30 in piglets
(unilateral irradiation)

Lethality	γ (^{60}Co)	n + γ (Silene reactor)	
(percent)	Total mid-line tissue dose (Gy)	total mid-line tissue dose (Gy)	partial mid-line tissue dose (Gy)
100	9.8	5.3-5.7	γ 2.9-3.1 n 2.4-2.6
		4.6-4.7	γ 2.5-2.6 n 2.1-2.2
83	--	3.9-4.0	γ 2.3 n 1.7
67	--	3.7-3.8	γ 2.1 n 1.6-1.7
58	5.0	--	--
50	4.0	--	--
33	--	3.1-3.4	γ 1.7-1.9 n 1.4-1.6

Clinical signs

In the range of total doses tested (3.1 to 9.8 Gy in mid-line tissue dose), for the two types of radiation fields the clinical signs correspond to behaviour, digestive and haemostasis disorders.

The liveliness of the piglets was more reduced when they received a higher dose. It was practically normal after 4 Gy gamma and 3.1 to 3.4 Gy neutrons + gammas. All the animals which were going to die within thirty days became prostrated 2 or 3 days before death and entered a deep coma in the last phase. In one experiment only (5.3 to 5.7 Gy neutrons + gamma) the behaviour was permanently upset from the end of exposure: the piglets were less active, seemed indifferent and did not react to care. This behaviour looks like Early Transient Incapacitation (ETI) pointed out by several authors after exposure with a high neutron component dose or after a very high dose of gamma-rays.

During the day following the exposure, appetite was irregular in most animals, all the more marked as the dose was higher. Sometimes the appetite disappeared completely. It was upset again during phases of diarrhoea and constipation. It disappeared shortly before death. Diarrhoea was noted during the first week. It culminated between day 3 and day 5 and was followed by a period of constipation. These digestive disorders were all the more noticeable, of greater duration and affected more piglets as the doses were higher.

Haemostatic disorders appeared after a certain delay. They were obvious in all animals (or almost, at the lowest doses: 4 Gy gamma and 3.1 to 3.4 Gy gamma + neutrons) by petechia which appeared between day 8 and day 11. Furthermore, at more or less the same time, the piglets which were to die before 30 days exhibited other haemorrhagic signs: epistaxis, haematuria, melaena, ocular haematoma, etc., of greater severity and duration as the doses were increased.

Lethality data

Death often took place at night and was caused by cardiac failure. Autopsy most often showed that the most serious lesion was diffuse haemorrhage of the myocardium. The carcass, which was extremely anaemic, especially showed signs of haemorrhage in one or several organs, often including the diaphragm, the intestines, the kidneys and the bladder. No signs of infection were apparent. Figure 2 shows the cumulative mortality rate after each of the doses and shows that generally mortality began during the second week and, when the dose was lower, lasted a longer period of time and involved a smaller number of animals.

166

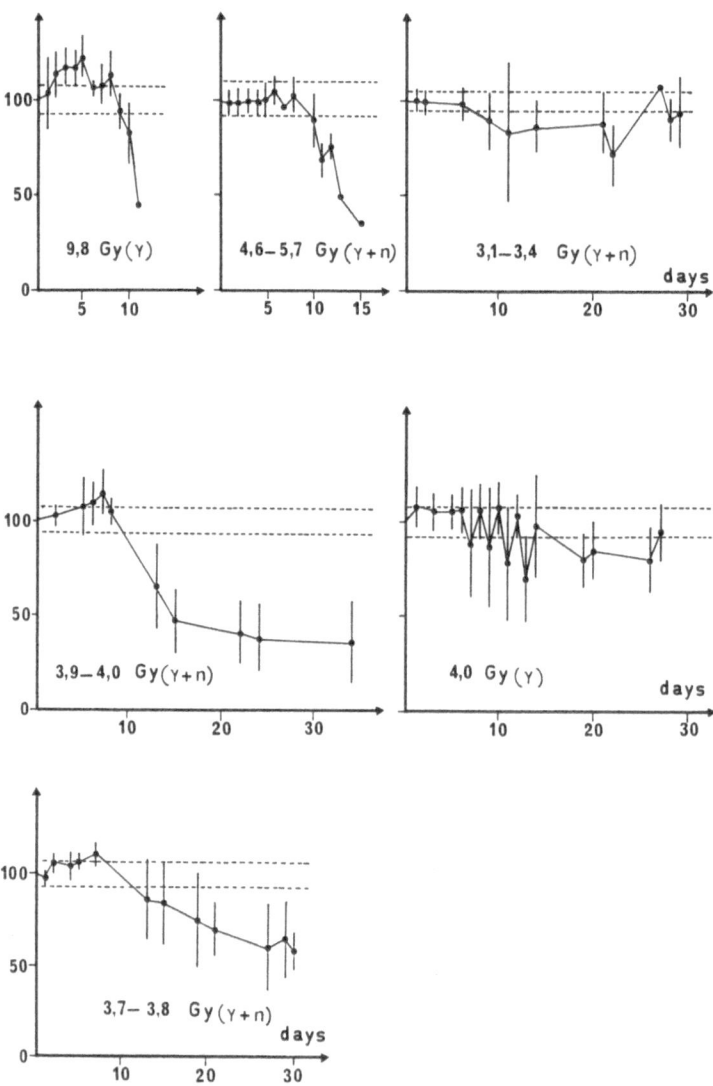

Figure 3: Evolution of erythrocytes in pigs after unilateral irradiation, The doses are expressed as tissue dose free-in-air.

Blood data

The result of each cell count is the average of 6 measurements (3 by sample) but only one white leucocyte and one reticulocyte count were established for each piglet and each day of observation. For reasons of individual variation, these are standardized by referring them to the values found before exposure for the animal under consideration. Figures 3 to 7 show the average values by groups of animals of these standardized ratios and their standard deviation. Variations observed in the control are also given.

At LD 100 (9.8 Gy gamma and at least 4.6 Gy neutron and gamma) the ratios of red cell counts vary very little for 8 to 9 days, and then drop rapidly. It reached 60% of its initial value by the 10th to 11th day in pure gamma fluence, 50% by the 13th day in mixed fluence (Figure 3). At lower doses this reduction takes place at about the same time but is all the less marked as the total dose is lower. It is however greater in mixed fluence than in pure gamma fluence (60% versus 20%) at the same total dose of 4 Gy.

The number of leucocytes decreases rapidly after exposure and after 5 to 6 days reaches a very low level, all the lower as the dose is higher (Figure 4). In the animals which survive up to the 30th day this level rises again, but more slowly after exposure in neutron and gamma fluence than after exposure to gamma radiation only.

Compared to the number of leucocytes, the number of blood platelets decreases less rapidly, but by the 10th day reaches very low levels even after doses resulting in a reduced rate of lethality (Figure 5). Among the surviving piglets it tends to increase after 3 weeks but by the 30th day after a total dose of 4 Gy it does not exceed 10% of its initial value when exposure involved neutrons.

The available values show that the proportion of lymphocytes collapses in the first two days and returns to normal in the two following days (Figure 6), and that of reticulocytes develops in the same way but less rapidly (Figure 7): the minimum is reached at about the 5th day and the return to the initial values around the 10th day.

Discussion and conclusion

There is a convergence of clinical and haematological observations and of those made at autopsy. The piglets of 16 to 20 kg which received total doses (mid-line tissue dose) from 4 to 9.8 Gy in pure gamma fluence and from 3.1 to 5.7 Gy in mixed neutron + gamma fluence exhibited essentially the hematopoietic form of the acute radiation syndrome. The intestinal effect was confined to early diarrhoea, then constipation, fairly restrained and all the less as the total dose was lower.

The bone-marrow effect quickly exhibits severe leucopenia and especially, within a week, severe thrombocytopenia leading to spontaneous haemorrhages in most organs which, with subsequent aneamia, leads to death in the second ten-day period.

168

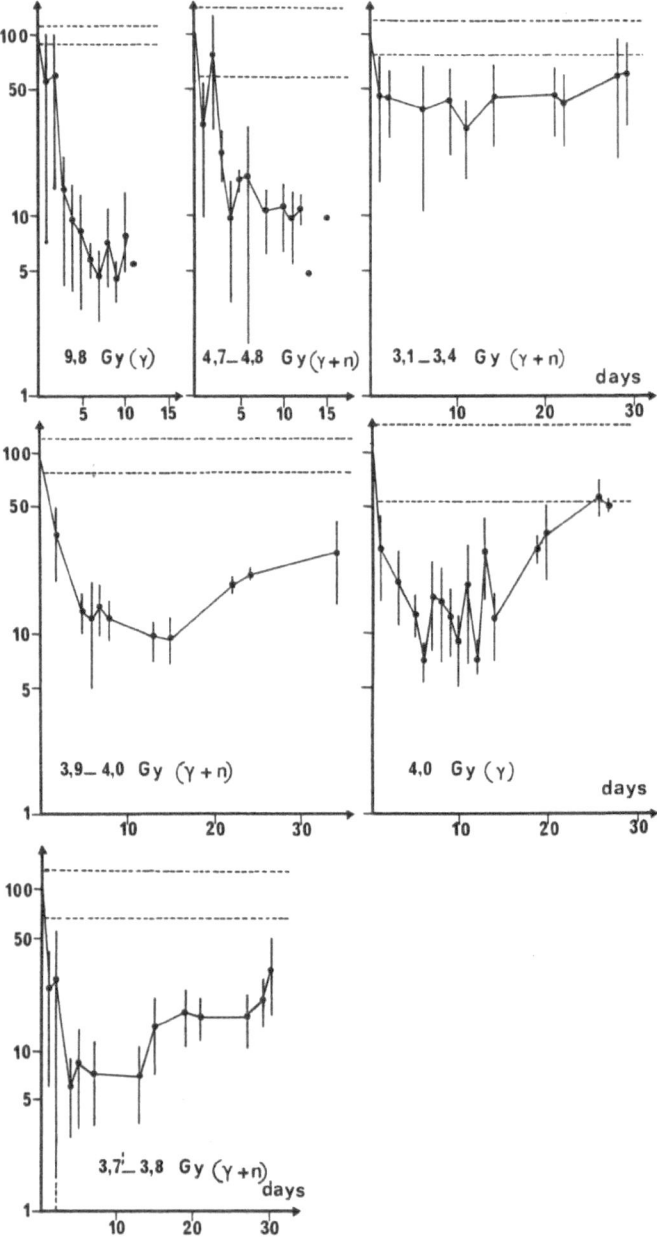

Figure 4: Evolution of leucocytes in pigs after unilateral irradiation. The doses are expressed as mid-line tissue dose free-in-air.

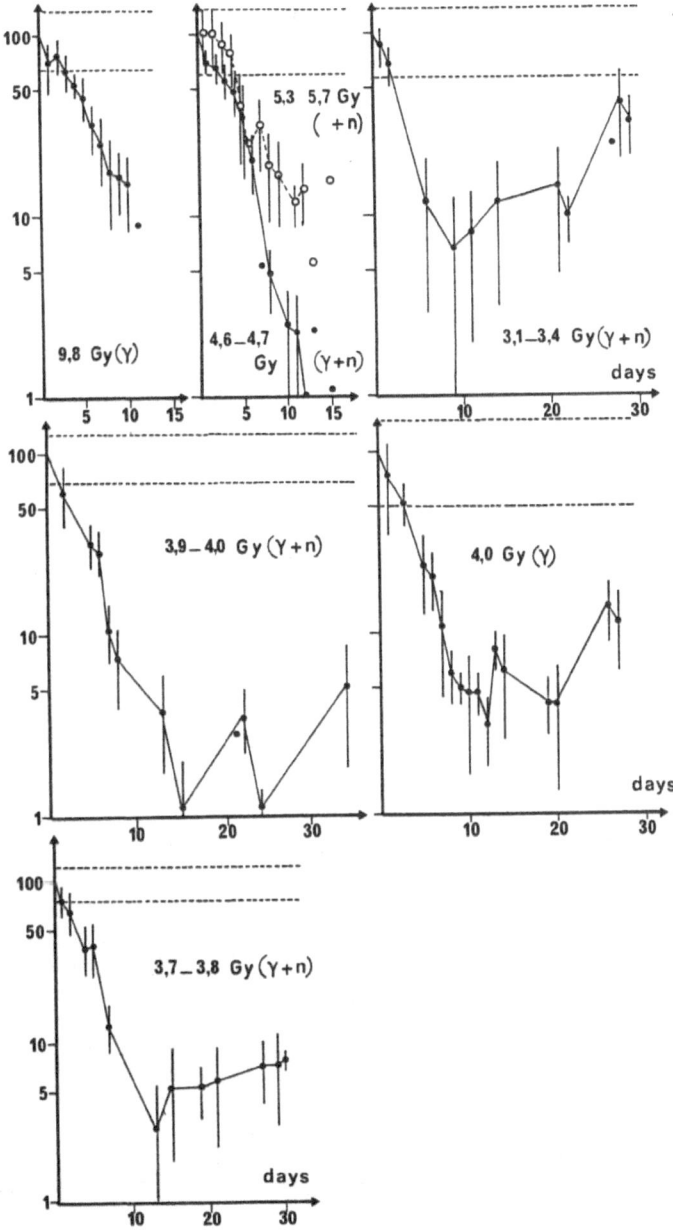

Figure 5: Evolution of thrombocytes in pigs after unilateral irradiation. The doses are expressed as tissue dose free-in-air

170

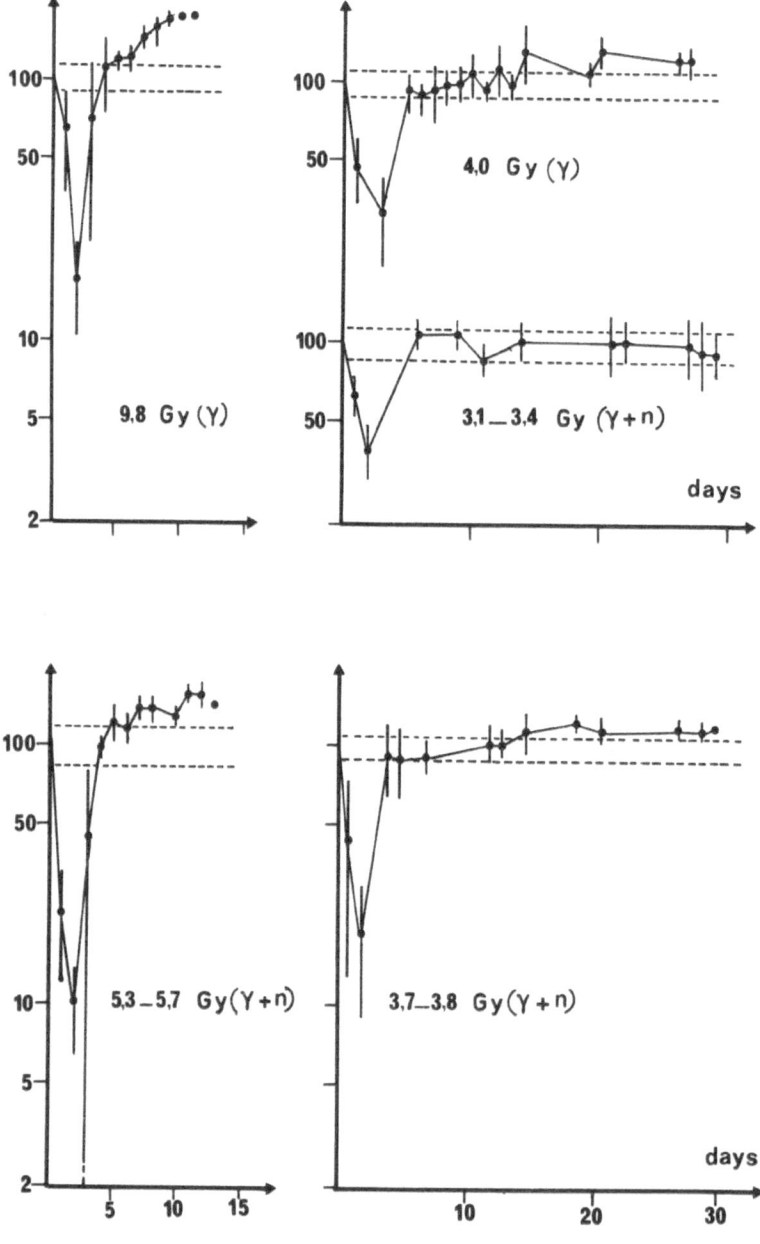

Figure 6: Evolution of lymphocytes in pigs after unilateral irradiation. The doses are expressed as tissue dose free-in-air.

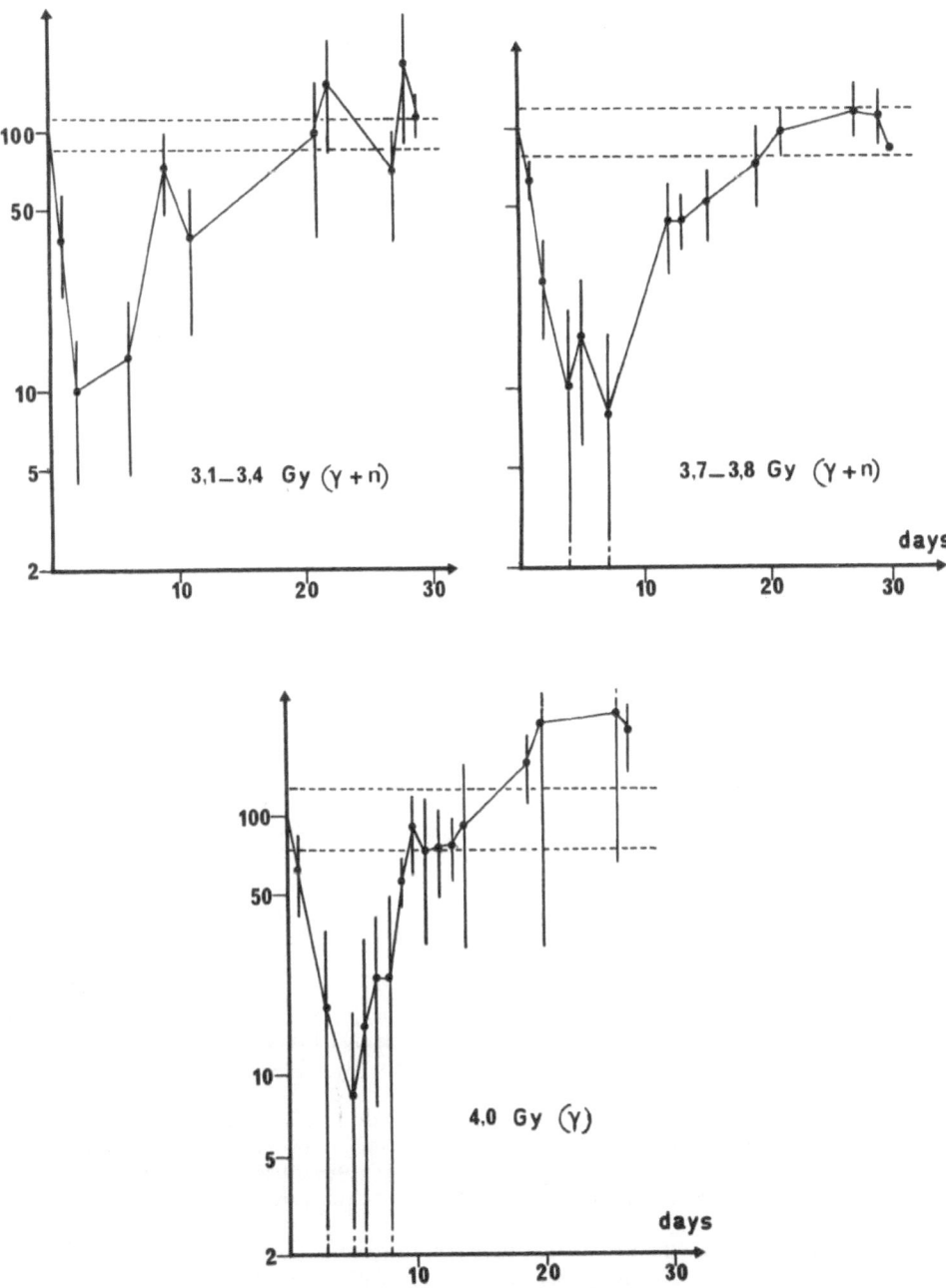

Figure 7: Evolution of reticulocytes in pigs after unilateral irradiation. The doses are expressed as tissue dose free-in-air.

In pure gamma fluence, the reduction of the dose from 9.8 to 4 Gy results in the diminution of these effects, the reduction of mortality from 100 to 50% and the lenghtening of its appearance delay from 10 to 23 days.

In mixed fluence (neutron + gamma), the total doses of 5.3 to 5.7 and 4.6 to 4.7 Gy have the same results from the clinical, haematological and mortality points of view as the dose of 9.8 Gy gamma radiation only. At a total dose of around 4 Gy, the mixed fluence is much more noxious than the pure gamma fluence.

For the dose range investigated our results agree with the data in the literature on gamma irradiation of large mammals, especially swine (4, 15, 16). They also agree with findings on monkeys, rats and humans where the thrombocyte rate reaches its minimum around the 10th day after exposure. The same clinical and haematological signs were exhibited by monkeys irradiated in the same way.

Our results differ from the data found in the literature in the value of the RBE of neutrons in large mammals (1-5, 17). We found the value greater than 1.0 even when taking such an unfit reference as the mid-line tissue dose.

Studies undertaken elsewhere on dosimetry in phantoms of swine should allow a better knowledge of neutron + gamma bone-marrow doses in each medullary area, and thus specify the relative survival of marrow cells, the role of which is the main point in moderating the effects of the hematopoietic syndrome.

References

1. Ainsworth, E.J., Leong, G.F., Kendall, K. and Alpen, E.L. Comparative lethality response of neutron and X irradiated dogs: Influence of dose rate and exposure aspect. Radiat.Res. 26, 32-43 (1965).

2. Alpen, E.L., Schil, O.S. and Tochilin, E. The effects of total body irradiation of dogs wit simulated fission neutrons. Radiat.Res. 12, 237-250 (1960).

3. Bond, V.P. , Carter, R.E., Robertson, J.S., Seymour, P.A. and Hechter, H.H. The effects of total body irradiation after fast neutron irradiation in dogs. Radiat.Res. 4, 139-153 (1956).

4. Wade jr., L. and Brown, D.G. LD50 (30) and dose distribution studies in swine irradiated with fission neutrons, 14 MeV neutrons and ^{60}Co gamma rays. In: Neutrons in Radiobiology, Oak Ridge, Conference November 1969. pp. 116-128, ntis, Springfield, (1970).

5. Mobley, T.S., De Feo, T.C. Cobalt-60 gamma irradiation of sheep: correlation of sixty-day median lethal studies with selected biochemical, hematologic and pathologic findings. Air Force Weapons Laboratory Report AFWL-TR-68-63 (1968).

6.   Otto, F.J. and Pfeiffer, U. Mortality response of mice after whole
     body exposure to 1,7- 5 MeV neutrons and X rays. Radiat.Res. $\underline{50}$,
     125-135 (1972).

7.   Corp, M.J., Hulse, E.V. and Batchelor, A.L. The RBE of fission
     neutrons, ^{60}Co gamma rays and 250 kV X rays for 28 day mortality in
     Syrian hamster. Int.J.Rad.Biol. $\underline{25}$, 61-66 (1974).

8.   Broerse, J.J., Bellum, D.W., Hollander, C.J. and Davids, J.A.G.
     Mortality of monkeys after exposure to fission neutrons and the
     effect of autologus bone marrow transplantation. Int.J.Rad.Biol.
     $\underline{34}$, 253-264 (1978).

9.   Carsten, A.L., Bond, V.P. and Thompson, K.R. The RBE of different
     energy neutrons as measured by the haematopoietic spleen-colony
     technique. Int.J.Rad.Biol. $\underline{29}$, 65-70 (1976).

10. Phillips, T.L. and Fu, K.K. Biological effects of 15 MeV neutrons.
     Int.J.Rad.Oncol.Biol.Phys. $\underline{1}$, 1139-1147 (1976).

11. Hall. E.J. The relative effectiveness of californium 252. In: Some
     physical, dosimetry and biomedical aspects of californium 252.
     Karlsruhe, 14-18 April 1975 (1976), pp. 151-161. International Ato-
     mic Energy Agency, Vienna (1978).

12. Lemaire, G., Maas, J. and Grillon, G. Les cellules germinales, un
     modele dans l'analyse des facteurs EBR des neutrons de fission aux
     faibles doses tant en irradiation aigue qu'en irradiation
     chronique. In: Fourth Symposium on neutron dosimetry, Munich-
     Neuherberg, EUR 7448, Vol. 1., pp. 185-197, Commission of European
     Communities, Luxembourg (1982).

13. Quantitative Concepts and Dosimetry in Radiobiology, ICRU report
     30. International Commission in Radiation Units and Measurements,
     Washington, 1979.

14. Ricourt, A., Van Dat, Medioni, R. and Perrier, J.C. Campagne
     Internationale d'intercomparaison sur la dosimetrie neutronique
     faite au TNO et au GSF (Octobre-Novembre 1975). Commissariat à
     l'Energie Atomique, Rapport CEA-R-4793 (1976).

15. Chambers jr., F.W., Biles, C.R., Bodenlos, L.J. and Dowling, J.H.
     Mortality and clinical signs in swine exposed to total body
     cobalt-60 gamma irradiation. Radiat.Res. $\underline{22}$, 316-333 (1964).

16. Vaiman, M. Guenet, J.L., Maas, J. and Nizza, P. Etude clinique et
     symtomatologique chez le porc soumis à une radiation gamma totale à
     dose létale. Commisariat à l'Energie Atomique, Rapport CEA-R-3001
     (1966).

17. Brown, D.G. and Haywood, F.F. 14 MeV neutron irradiation of swine:
     dosimetry and clinical response. Health Phys. $\underline{24}$, 627-636 (1973).

THE OCCURRENCE OF RADIATION SYNDROMES IN RODENTS AND
MONKEYS IN DEPENDENCE ON DOSE RATE AND
RADIATION QUALITY

J.J. Broerse and J. Zoetelief
Radiobiological Institute TNO, Rijswijk, The Netherlands

Introduction

The nature of radiation syndromes as well as the survival time following whole body irradiation are dependent on the absorbed dose. For
doses in excess of several, Gy animals can die due to failure of haemopoiesis; death is observed between 10 and 20 days after irradiation. At
increasing dose levels, in excess of 6 to 8 Gy, mortality is caused by
irreversible damage to the gastro-intestinal tract; death occurs within
approximately 6 days. The effectiveness of different types of radiation
can be derived from the LD_{50} values for the occurrence of the two syndromes in monkeys, rats and mice as reported in the present contribution. Techniques, such as the spleen colony assay and the microscopic
scoring of surviving intestinal crypt stem cells have made it possible
to investigate the cellular effects inducing the clinical syndromes.

The survival of haemopoietic and intestinal crypt stem cells in
mice is presented for irradiations with photons and neutrons of different energies. Values for the relative biological effectiveness (RBE)
derived from cell survival curves are correlated with those obtained
from the LD_{50} studies.

Protraction or fractionation of the irradiation will reduce the
severity of the biological effect due to various biological mechanisms.
The effects of dose rate will be exemplified with studies in mice.

LD_{50} after photon and neutron irradiation

Information about the clinical symptoms associated with the occurrence of the bone marrow and gastro-intestinal syndromes can be found
elsewhere (Bond et al. 1965, Vriesendorp and van Bekkum 1980). The 50
percent mortality of the animals within the period of 7 to 20 days after
irradiation can be taken as an endpoint for the induction of the bone
marrow syndrome ($LD_{50/30d}$). As indicated in figure 1 for X-irradiations
of Rhesus monkeys an LD_{50} of 5.25 Gy is observed and the animals can be
rescued by an autologous bone marrow transplantation up to doses of
approximately 9 Gy. Above this dose level the monkeys die due to a
delayed intestinal syndrome (Broerse et al. 1978). For irradiation of
Rhesus monkeys with fission neutrons an LD_{50} of approximately 2.6 Gy is
observed. The autologous bone marrow transplantation is effective in
protecting the animals from haemopoietic death after neutron irradiation
up to a total dose of 5 Gy. For neutrons, the dose values quoted refer
to total absorbed dose averaged over the monkey.

Dose mortality studies in mice show a similar pattern. In figure 2
studies on 30-day mortality and 5-day mortality in F-1 hybrid mouse are

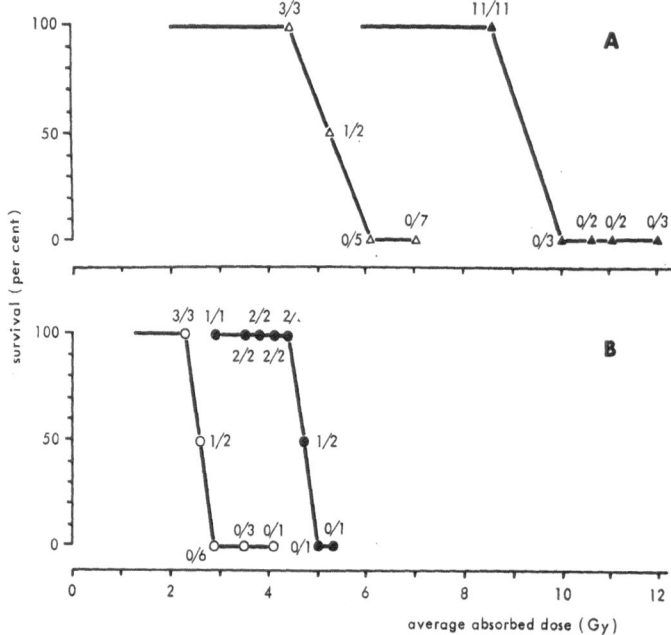

Figure 1   The survival of monkeys within 30 days after irradiation
with 300 kV X rays (part A) and fission neutrons (part B)
for control animals (open symbols) and animals treated with
autologous bone marrow (closed symbols). At each dose
level the number of surviving animals and the total number
irradiated is given (Broerse et al. 1978).

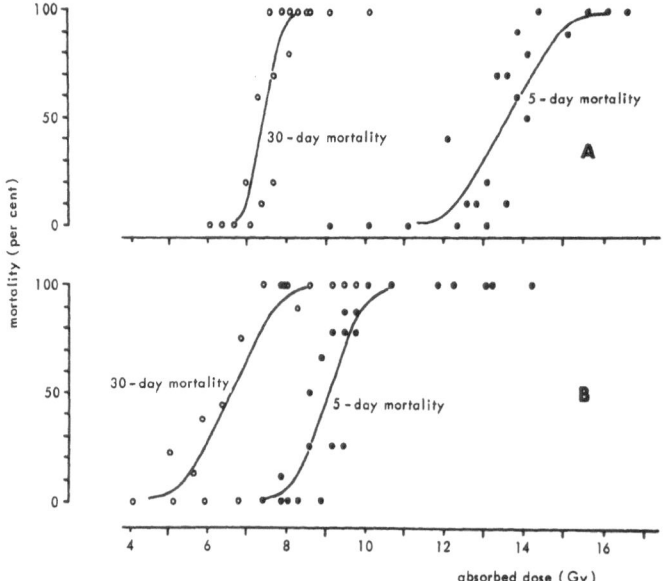

Figure 2   Mortality of (CBA x C57Bl)F_1 mice either within 30 days or
within 5 days after irradiation with X rays (part A) or 15
MeV neutrons (part B) (Broerse 1969).

Table I

LD $_{50/30d}$ (in Gy) after 300 kV X- and ^{137}Cs γ-irradiation
for both sexes in various mouse strains available at TNO

strain	300 kV X rays	^{137}Cs γ rays	300 kV X rays	^{137}Cs γ rays
	Female		Male	
Balb/C	5.3	6.4	5.4	6.1
Nude	-	-	-	6.4
ND2	6.1	6.9	-	7.1
RFO	6.4	-	5.9	-
C3H	6.5	7.4	6.2	7.3
AKR	6.5	7.6	6.2	7.1
C57 bl/ka	6.2	7.7	6.2	7.7
RFM	6.6	-	6.3	-
C57 bl/Rij	6.5	7.9	6.4	7.4
CBA/Rij	6.7	7.2	6.7	7.5
CBA/T6	6.7	7.5	6.7	7.6
SJL/J	-	7.7	-	7.7
BC3	-	8.1	-	7.7
R57	7.1	-	6.7	-
BCBA/F1	7.1	8.0	6.8	7.9
GRS	7.3	-	6.8	-
DBA2	-	8.4	-	8.1
CD2	7.1	8.7	6.9	8.2

The uncertainty is 3 per cent at a 68 per cent confidence level

Table II

$LD_{50/30}$ (in Gy) after 300 kV X-irradiation
of both sexes in various rat strains
available at TNO

strain	female	male
Choco	4.5	-
Glaxo	5.0	5.4
Wag Rij	5.5	6.0
Brown Norway	5.9	6.4
Sprague Dawley	6.9	7.4
Brofo	7.8	8.0

The uncertainty is about 3 percent at a 68 percent confidence level.

summarized, for irradiation with X rays and 15 MeV neutrons produced
by the d+T reaction (Broerse 1969). The 5-day mortality in mice can be
taken as a criterion for the occurrence of the gastro-intestinal syndrome ($LD_{50/5d}$). In tables I and II the $LD_{50/30d}$ values for respectively
mice and rats (generally irradiated at an age of about 12 weeks) used
at the Radiobiological Institute TNO are summarized. It should be noted
that for the same species considerable differences in radiosensitivity are
observed. The $LD_{50/30d}$ values after X irradiaton vary from 5.3 to 7.3
Gy for different mouse strains and from 4.5 to 8.0 Gy for rats. The
differences in sensitivity between the two sexes are generally marginal.
The gamma rays of ^{137}Cs have a lower effectiveness than 300 kV X
rays. An average RBE of 0.86 is observed for gamma radiation.

It can be concluded from figures 1 and 2 that the intervals between the LD_{50} values for the occurrence of bone marrow and intestinal
syndromes are smaller for neutrons than for X rays. However, for photon and neutron irradiation of monkeys and mice the bone marrow syndrome is observed at lower dose values than the gastro-intestinal syndrome. This implies that bone marrow transplantation can be of benefit
for survival after an accidental irradiation with neutrons as well as with
photons. For total body irradiation of dogs, Vriesendorp and van
Bekkum (1980) observed an $LD_{50/30d}$ of 3.7 Gy. In addition they found
a linear relationship between the number of bone marrow cells required
for 50 percent rescue and the body weight of different species.

Calculated on the basis of the LD_{50} values, the relative biological
effectiveness (RBE) of 15 MeV neutrons for induction of the bone marrow syndrome and the gastro-intestinal syndrome in mice is equal to 1.1
and 1.4, respectively. For the Hammersmith neutron beam, with a mean

energy of 7 MeV produced by the d(16)+Be reaction, the RBE for the bone marrow and the intestinal syndrome in mice is equal to 1.5 and 2.3, respectively (Hornsey et al. 1965). For fission neutrons, with a mean energy of 1 MeV the RBE values for the two radiation syndromes in CBA mice are equal to 1.9 and 3.0 (Davids 1970). The relative biological effectiveness for the two radiation syndromes as a function of the neutron energy is summarized in figure 3 in comparison with values obtained for survival of human kidney cells (Broerse 1974). The increase in RBE with decreasing neutron energy is in agreement with other studies which show maximum RBE values for neutron energies of approximately 0.5 to 1.0 MeV.

On the basis of the $LD_{50/30d}$ values of 5.25 Gy for X rays and 2.6 Gy for fission neutrons the RBE for the occurrence of the bone marrow syndrome in monkeys is approximately 2. It should be stressed that the value for the neutron irradiation is expressed as total absorbed dose. Considering the different efficiency of the contaminating gamma component (24 percent of the total absorbed dose) relative to the neutron component, an RBE of approximately 2.4 can be derived for the neutron component only. It is rather difficult to provide information about the RBE for the occurrence of the intestinal syndrome since the survival time due to intestinal damage after X irradiation could be prolonged by good clinical care of the animals (Broerse et al. 1978).

Influence of dose rate

When the delivery of the absorbed dose is protracted over periods in excess of one hour a number of processes including cellular repair, cell synchronization and cell multiplication will reduce the severity of the biological effect. In figure 4 iso-effect curves for $LD_{50/30d}$ in different mouse strains after total body irradiation with X rays are summarized. The curves show a progressive increase with exposure time with a trend to level off for times longer than 6 to 8 hours (Dutreix et al. 1982). A similar tendency has been observed for the occurrence of bone marrow syndrome and intestinal syndrome in mice after continuous irradiation with ^{137}Cs gamma radiation (Broerse 1969). It can be concluded from figure 5 that for photon irradiation the intestinal cells show a higher capacity for recovery then the haemopoietic cells. It is anticipated that these differences in repair of sublethal damage are related to the shapes of the survival curves of the stem cells involved.

Effects at the cellular level

The radiation syndromes involve a number of clinical disorders including haemorrhages, infections, and loss of fluids and electrolytes. It should be stressed, however, that the primary cause of the radiation syndromes lies in effects at the cellular level i.e. the survival of haemopoietic and intestinal crypt stem cells. Survival of the haemopoietic stem cells can be investigated with the spleen colony technique introduced by Till and McCulloch (1961). Information on the survival of bone marrow stem cells for in vitro and in vivo irradiations after single dose and fractionated irradiations with X rays and 15 MeV neutrons can be found elsewhere (Broerse et al. 1971). For the single dose irradiation with 300 kV X rays a D_o value of 0.73 Gy and an extrapolation number of 2.5 was observed.

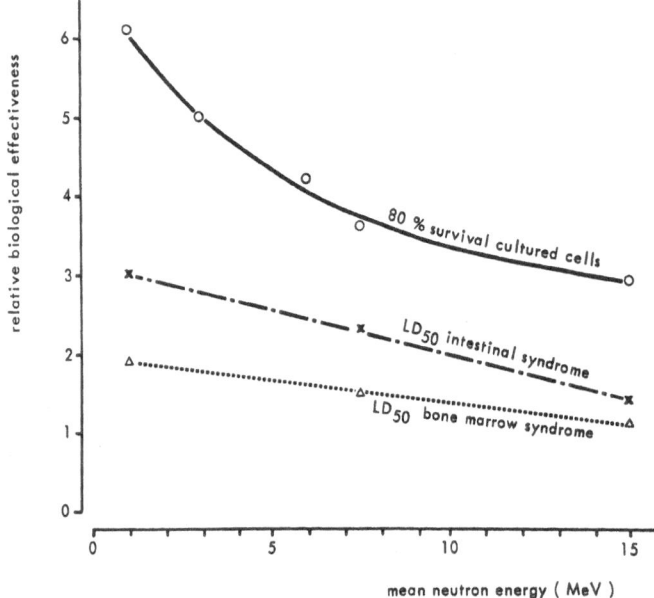

Figure 3   RBE as a function of mean neutron energy for survival of
cultured cells at low doses and for induction of intestinal
and haemopoietic syndromes in mice (Broerse 1974).

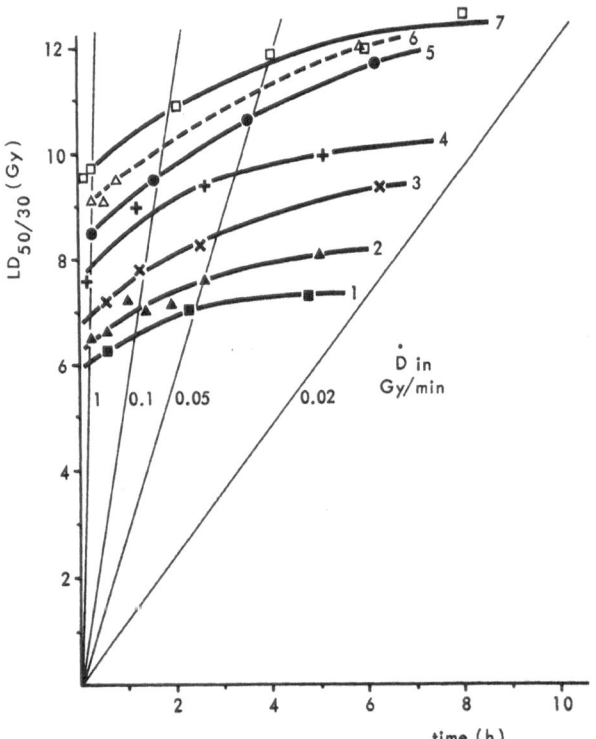

Figure 4   Isoeffect curves as a function of exposure time observed in
different mouse strains (curves 1 to 7) for $LD_{50/30d}$ after
continuous irradiation (Dutreix et al 1982).

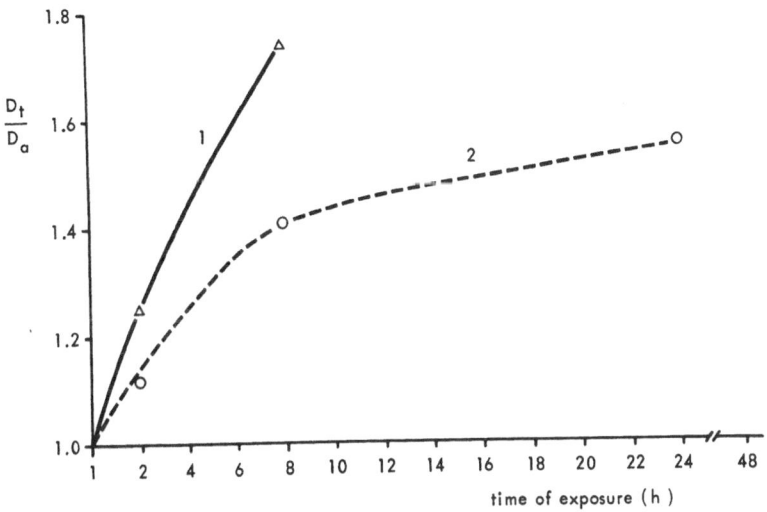

Figure 5   The ratio of the LD_{50} for protracted irradiation (D_t) to the LD_{50} for acute irradiation (D_a) as a function of exposure time. Curve 1 corresponds to intestinal death, curve 2 to haemopoietic death.

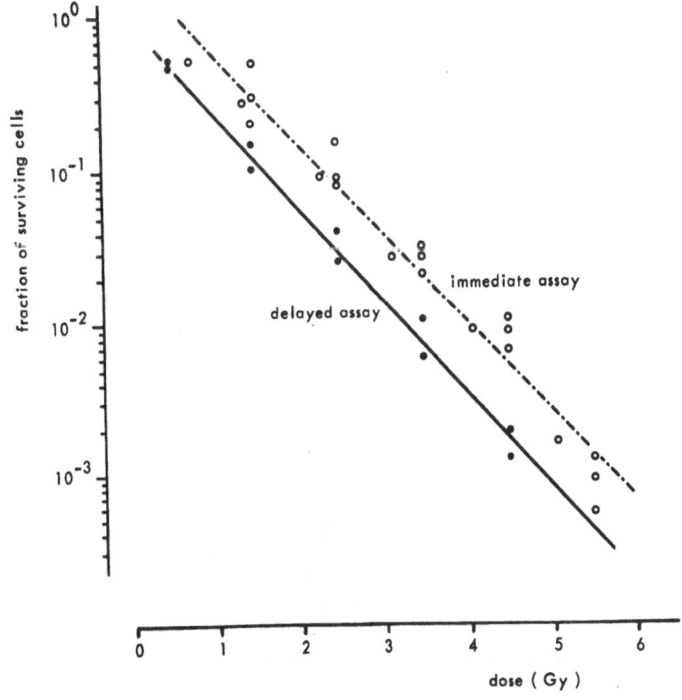

Figure 6   Survival of haemopoietic stem cells in the femora of mice after single dose in vivo irradiation with 300 kV X rays determined with immediate and delayed assay (van Putten et al. 1970).

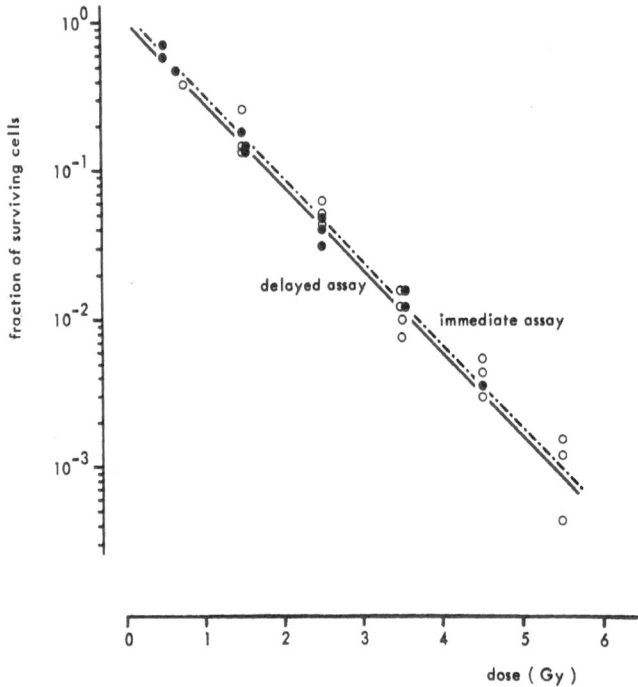

Figure 7 Survival of haemopoietic stem cells in mice after *in vivo* irradiation with 15 MeV neutrons determined with immediate and delayed assay (van Putten et al. 1970).

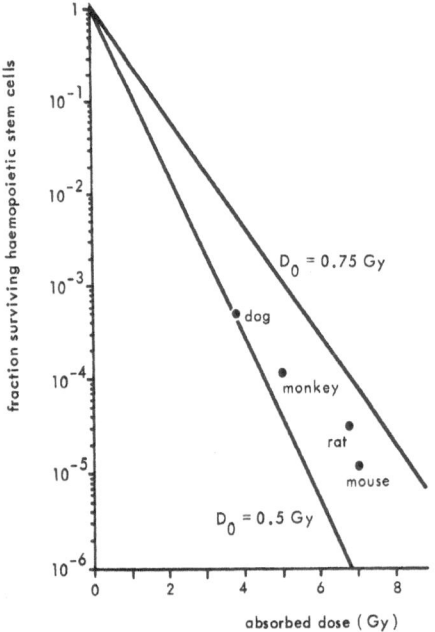

Figure 8 Estimation of survival of haemopoietic stem cells in different species (Vriesendorp and van Bekkum 1980).

Studies on the survival of colony forming units (CFU) in mouse bone marrow after fractionated irradiation showed a slightly higher effectiveness for X rays than for fast neutrons i.e. the RBE of 15 MeV neutrons is smaller than 1 for these experimental conditions (van Putten et al. 1970). This result is unexpected in view of the small shoulder in the survival curve for single dose irradiation with 15 MeV neutrons and the smaller repair which is usually observed in split-dose irradiations in comparison with X rays. A partial explanation for this observation was obtained from another series of experiments on the effect of single doses of neutrons and X rays in which a delay of 24 hours was allowed between irradiation and sacrifice of the donors for assay (van Putten et al. 1970). As shown in figure 6 the delayed assay causes a marked reduction in colony forming cells from the bone marrow of X-irradiated mice. This phenomenon of loss of CFU did not occur for the neutron irradiation (see figure 7). It seems most likely that the loss of CFU after X-irradiation is caused by differentiation of colony-forming cells to a cell type which has lost the capability for proliferation to the size of a visible spleen colony (van Putten et al. 1970). However, there is no explanation for the absence of this phenomenon after neutron irradiation. Differences in the effect of delayed assay imply that X rays can be slightly more effective in fractionated irradiations than neutrons. In consequence the RBE for immediate assay will be higher than the RBE for delayed assay and for fractionated exposures. The studies on CFU survival indicate that in addition to differences in repair of sublethal damage for X and neutron irradiation, differences in other biological mechanisms will determine the overall effectiveness after fractionated exposures. The interpretation of these qualitative differences will require additional information on the population kinetics of the stem cells after X and neutron irradiation.

Vriesendorp and van Bekkum (1980) analysed the fractional survival of haemopoietic stem cells at the LD_{50} values for total body irradiation in different species. Their analysis shown in figure 8 predicts D_o values of between 0.5 and 0.75 Gy for all haemopoietic stem cells.

For a valid comparison of the effects of neutron and X-irradiation on the intact animal and the effects on the haemopoietic stem cells, comparable survival levels should be considered. Doses in the $LD_{50/30d}$ range correspond to surviving fractions between 10^{-3} and 10^{-4}. At a surviving fraction of 10^{-3} the RBE of 15 MeV neutrons for single dose in vivo irradiation is 1.03 which is not significantly different from the RBE of 1.1 for the occurrence of the bone marrow syndrome. Somewhat larger RBE values have been observed for CFU survival after irradiation with collimated d+T neutrons (Broerse et al. 1971). This difference has to be attributed to the presence of low energy neutrons produced by the collimator.

The survival of intestinal crypt stem cells has been determined by scoring the number of regenerating crypts (microcolonies) in the jejunum of the mouse (Withers and Elkind 1970). The survival curves for jejunal crypt stem cells in mice show D_o values of 1.67 Gy and 1.4 Gy for X rays and 15 MeV neutrons, respectively. An RBE value of 1.4 can be calculated at radiation doses in the lethal range for these mice.

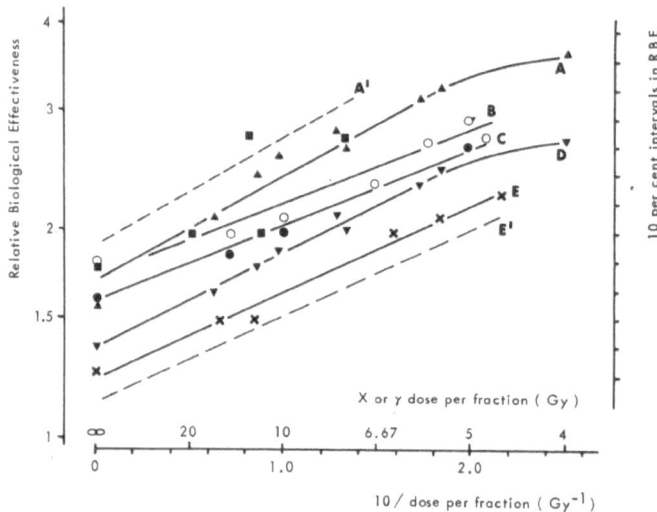

Figure 9   RBE for survival of intestinal crypt stem cells as a function
of the photon dose per fraction for various neutron beams.
Curve A: d(16)+Be neutrons, curve A': same results after
modification to common dose standard, curve B: collimated d+T
neutrons, curve C: collimated d+T neutrons at 10 cm depth,
curve D: d(50) + Be neutrons, curve E: uncollimated d+T
neutrons, curve E': same results after modification to common
dose standard (Hendry and Greene, 1976).

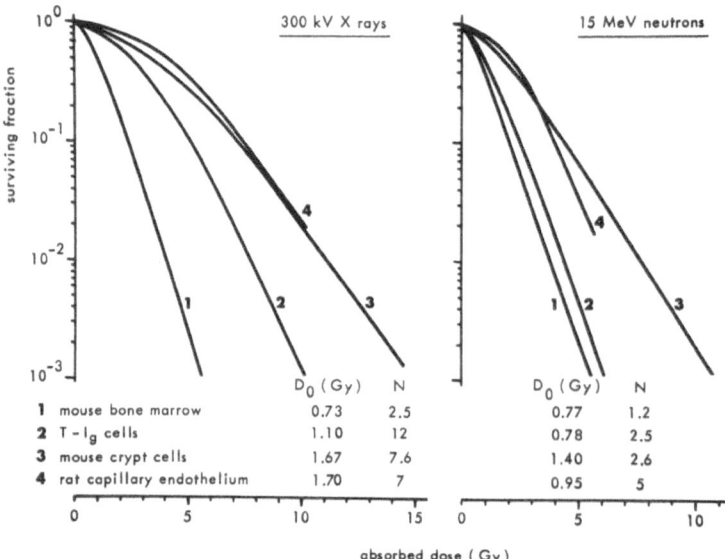

Figure 10 Survival curves of clonogenic cells in different types of
normal tissues (Broerse et al. 1977) and parameters fitted
according to: $S(D)/S(O) = 1- \left[1- \exp (-D/D_o) \right]^N$.

This value is in good agreement with the RBE for the $LD_{50/5d}$. The intestinal microcolony assay has been used by various groups to determine the RBE for different neutron beams (see e.g. Hendry and Greene, 1976). The RBE values as a function of the photon dose per fraction for d(16)+Be, d+T and d(50)+Be neutrons are summarized in figure 9. The highest RBE values are observed for smaller doses per fraction and generally also for the lower neutron energies. The RBE values for collimated d+T neutron beams are higher than for irradiations free in air without collimator. In accordance with these findings Zywietz et al (1979) observed an RBE of 2.1 for survival of intestinal crypt stem cells after irradiation with the collimated d+T neutron beam at Hamburg.

A summary of survival curves of different types of clonogenic cells is shown in figure 10 (Broerse et al. 1977). The results clearly indicate that a considerable variation of intrinsic radiosensitivity exists for X rays: bone marrow stem cells being the most sensitive and intestinal stem cells rather resistant. It can further be concluded that similar but somewhat smaller differences are observed for irradiation with 15 MeV neutrons.

Conclusions

1. Among the various cell populations, bone marrow stem cells are the most sensitive . Exposure of different animal species to doses of X rays between 4 and 8 Gy will produce the haemopoietic syndrome. There are no long term acting prophylactic agents available to prevent the lethal consequences of severe bone marrow damage. The only way to rescue animals from lethal exposure in the lower dose range is to apply a bone marrow transplantation.

2. Even within the same species (e.g. mice and rats) considerable variations are observed in $LD_{50/30d}$ values after photon irradiation. Gamma radiation has a lower effectiveness than 300 kV X rays, the RBE for the occurrence of the haemapoietic syndrome is generally around 0.86.

3. The RBE values for the occurrence of radiation syndromes depend on the neutron energy. For different animal species, RBE values between 1.1 and 2.4 have been observed for bone marrow syndrome and between 1.4 and 3 for the intestinal syndrome.

4. RBE values observed for occurrence of radiation syndromes are in good agreement with those for effects on bone marrow and intestinal crypt stem cells.

5. It should be emphasized that the RBE values reported in this paper refer to total body irradiation in which all possible measures are taken to achieve homogeneous irradiation. For irradiations with inhomogeneous distribution of the absorbed dose over the animal (e.g. partial body exposure) appreciable variations in biological response are to be anticipated.

References

Bond V.P., Fliedner, T.M. and Archambeau, J.V. 1965 Mammalian Radiation Lethality (New York: Academic Press).

Broerse J.J. 1969, Dose-mortality studies for mice irradiated with X-rays, gamma-rays and 15 MeV neutrons. Int.J.Radiat.Biol, 15, 115.

Broerse J.J. 1974, Review of RBE values of 15 MeV neutrons for effects on normal tissues. Europ.J.Cancer 10, 225

Broerse J.J., Engels A.C., Lelieveld P. Putten L.M. van, Duncan W, Greene D., Massey J.B., Gilbert C.W., Hendry J.H., and Howard A., 1971, The survival of colony-forming units in mouse bone marrow after in vivo irradiation with D-T neutrons, X- and gamma-radiation. Int.J.Radiat.Biol., 19, 101

Broerse J.J., Barendsen G.W., Freriks G. and Putten L.M. van, 1971, RBE values of 15 MeV neutrons for effects on normal tissues. Europ.J.Cancer. 7, 171.

Broerse J.J., Barendsen G.W., Gaiser J.F. and Zoetelief J., 1977. The importance of differences in intrinsic cellular radiosensitivity for the effectiveness of neutron radiotherapy treatments. In: Radiobiological Research and Radiotherapy (Vienna: International Atomic Energy Agency) II, 19.

Broerse J.J., Bekkum D.W. van, Hollander C.F. and Davids J.A.G., 1978. Mortality of monkeys after exposure to fission neutrons and the effect of autologous bone marrow transplantation. Int.J.Radiat. Biol. 34, 253

Davids J.A.G., 1970. Bone-marrow syndrome in CBA mice exposed to fast neutrons of 1.0 MeV mean energy. Effect of syngeneic bone-marrow transplantation. Int.J.Radiat.Biol. 17, 878

Dutreix J., Gluckman E., Brule J.M., 1982. Biological problems of total body irradiation. J.Eur.Radiother. 3, 165

Hendry J.H., Greene D., 1976. Re-evaluation of published neutron RBE values for mouse intestine. Brit.J,Radiol., 49, 195

Hornsey S., Vatistas S., Bewley D.K. and Parnell C.J., 1965. The effect of fractionation on four-day survival of mice after whole-body neutron irradiation. Brit.J.Radiol. 38, 878.

Putten L.M. van, Lelieveld P. and Broerse J.J., 1970. Effects of 300 kV X-rays and 15 MeV neutrons in single and fractionated doses on hemopoietic stem cells in mouse bone marrow. In: Proc. Conf. Time and Dose Relationships in Radiation Biology as Applied to Radiotherapy. (Springfield: NBS), 162

Till J.E. and McCulloch E.A., 1961. Direct measurement of radiation sensitivity of normal mouse bone marrow cells. Radiat Res. 14, 213.

Vriesendorp H.M. and Bekkum D.W. van, 1980. Role of total body irradiation in conditioning for bone marrow transplantation. In: Immunology of Bone Marrow Transplantation. (Berlin: Springer Verlag), 349.

Withers H.R. and Elkind M.M., 1970. Microcolony survival assay for cells of mouse intestinal mucosa exposed to radiation. Int.J.Radiat.Biol. 17, 261

Zijwietz F., Jung H., Hess A. and Franke H.I., 1979. Response of mouse intestine to 14 MeV neutrons. Int.J.Radiat.Biol. 35, 63.

THE RESPONSE OF MAN TO ACCIDENTAL IRRADIATION

K.F. BAVERSTOCK

MRC Radiobiology Unit, Harwell, Didcot, Oxon OX11 0RD
United Kingdom

Introduction

In the search for indications of the sensitivity of man to death
caused by bone marrow failure following exposure to whole-body
irradiation, those persons exposed in accidents with radiation are a
potentially useful source of information. Since most radiation
accidents occur in the work place, those exposed are clearly in normal
health and also, since such accidents are taken seriously by society,
there is likely to have been a very thorough investigation to establish
the extent of exposure of each exposed individual. On the other hand,
unplanned exposures by their very nature are bound to be a less reliable
source of information than experimental or other planned exposure, for
example during treatment by radiotherapy. In addition, those exposed
are likely to have been subject to some form of treatment following the
exposure which may or may not have been beneficial in terms of their
survival. Also, factors such as the distribution of dose within the
body, the dose rate, and the quality of the radiation may characterise a
particular accident limiting its general applicability. In fact nonuniformity of dose distribution and dose rate are known from animal
experiments to be so influential on sensitivity that it is probably best
to exclude from such assessments accidents in which the dose was not
uniformly distributed and for which the dose rate was not such that
exposure could be described as brief. By brief is meant a dose
delivered in a time scale short compared with that of cellular turnover.
Exposure to high LET radiations can be interpreted in terms of an
equivalent low LET dose by applying RBE values. As far as supportive
treatment following exposure is concerned it is possible to assess the
benefit gained and the possible influence on survival. Today there are
undoubtedly treatments which could make very considerable differences to
an irradiated individual's chances of survival, particularly if

precautions were taken prior to irradiation, but it is much more debatable whether the simple treatments available a decade or so ago were effective in more than making life more comfortable for the exposed victim.

With these thoughts in mind the accidents for which reasonably full published details are available were reviewed (Baverstock and Ash 1983). Of 16 accidents identified, only 2 were considered to be in the appropriate dose range, namely about 2-10 Gy, and to satisfy the conditions regarding uniformity of dose distribution and briefness of exposure. Both these accidents involved exposure to neutrons as well as to gamma rays, and therefore require interpretation in terms of a low LET equivalent dose. Additionally, since it is highly desirable that the dose be expressed in terms of absorbed dose to the bone marrow rather than, for example, as tissue kerma in air, the appropriate conversion has also to be carried out. In an appendix to their paper Baverstock and Ash (1983) considered in detail the dosimetries of these two accidents and the bearing these may have on the relevance of these accidents to the sensitivity of man to radiation-induced bone marrow failure.

The accidents

The accident at the Y12 plant at Oak Ridge, U.S.A. occurred during maintenance operations on a fuel reprocessing plant. The details are given in some detail in an official report of the accident (ORNL 1958) and by Hurst et al (1959). Briefly, uranyl nitrate solution from another part of the plant was inadvertantly allowed to collect in a steel drum close to where men were working. Eventually sufficient solution collected in the drum for a vigorous fission chain reaction to be initiated during which neutrons and gamma-rays were emitted. It seems highly probable that the initial reaction was short-lived (of the order of a fraction of a second) since gas generated from the radiolysis of the water quenched the reaction quickly. However, as soon as the bubbling died down and the critical geometry was regained, the reaction was reinitiated. There is uncertainty about the precise temporal distribution of the exposure in the first several seconds because the site radiation monitors recorded an offscale reading for some time, but later readings indicate that several pulses occurred, the intensity of which diminished with time. Alarms sounded within a few seconds of the initial burst of radiation and the area was quickly evacuated. It therefore seems probable that the first and probably by far the largest pulse of radiation gave rise to the greater part of the exposure to the personnel (ORNL 1958).

Following the accident there was a lengthy screening process to determine which personnel had been exposed. Eventually a number of men were identified from measurements made on indium foil badges and among these were seven thought to have received substantial doses, of the order of 1 Gy or more. In order to determine doses to individuals measurements of sodium-24 in blood were made for each exposed person and later a calibration experiment was carried out to relate this neutron induced activity in the body to the first collision dose[*] from neutrons. At the same time threshold measurements of the neutron spectrum and the neutron-to-gamma ratio were also made.

The second accident, at Vinca in Yugoslavia, involved an entirely different set of circumstances. The Institute at Vinca houses a research reactor moderated by heavy water. The assembly is unshielded and is normally operated at zero power. The accident occurred when the reactor ran temporarily out of control for a period of several minutes (IAEA 1961; Hurst et al 1961).

Once again the measurements of sodium-24 activity in blood were made on each exposed individual and a calibration experiment performed at which the measurements made were very similar to those made at Y12. There was, however, a marked difference between the qualities of the neutron spectra at the two accidents. The presence of D_2O in the Vinca reactor led to the emission of a very much 'softer' neutron spectrum than that at Y12. Relatively low energy neutrons, while not being very penetrating themselves do give rise to the so called auto-gamma dose, i.e. gamma-rays emitted after capture of neutrons with various atoms of which hydrogen is the most important in tissue. Because of this the two accidents are not comparable on a first collision dose basis and it is

---

[*]The first collision dose (FCD) is the dose to a small isolated volume of tissue in air at the position of the subject. It takes no account of attenuation due to tissues shielding the volume or of back scatter from deeper lying tissues. It is referred to often as the tissue dose free in air and approximates closely to tissue kerma in air.

therefore necessary to reassess the dosimetry in terms of absorbed dose to bone marrow.

Dosimetric reassessment

A close examination of the calibration experiments at both accidents reveals some cause for concern. For example, at the Y12 calibration experiment a burro rather than a phantom was exposed to the neutron fluence to determine the ratio between sodium-24 activation and neutron fluence. Since the relationship between these two parameters includes a term for the ratio of the projected area of the phantom in the beam (A) to its volume (V) (Delafield et al 1973), it is by no means certain that the burro will have been representative, in this respect, of man. At Vinca, plastic man-shaped phantoms were used but they were filled with a sodium chloride solution to represent tissue. For a solution of sodium chloride with a physiological concentration of sodium ions the chloride concentration will be far higher than that found in tissue. Since chlorine has a large cross-section for neutron interaction it seems possible that the extent of capture of neutrons by sodium in the phantom will not necessarily represent that to be expected in tissue.

Fortunately it has become possible to cross-check these calibration experiments using theoretically calculated relationships between sodium-24 activity and neutron fluence (Cross 1981) given that the energy spectrum for the neutrons is known. These calculations, given in detail in an appendix (Baverstock and Ash 1983), highlight the importance of knowing the orientation of the exposed individual in the neutron beam. The reason is that for a given individual the ratio of projected area in the beam to volume (A/V) can vary by more than a factor 2 depending upon whether exposure to the neutrons is from the front or rear (i.e. A-P or P-A) or from the side. Thus if exposure is from one aspect only and the orientation of the subject at the time of exposure is not known, the calculated first collision dose is bound to be uncertain by a factor nearly 2. The presence of neutrons scattered from the floors and walls adds an isotropic element to the exposure in practice which tends to reduce the observed ratio between frontal and lateral exposure (Cross 1981). If on the other hand exposure was from more than one aspect, an average value for A/V could be assumed although of course this does not necessarily remove all the uncertainty.

In the case of these two accidents it is worth considering in some detail what information regarding orientation can be gained from the detailed accounts of the accidents.

The circumstances of the Y12 accident point clearly to exposure being the result of pulses of radiation emitted from the drum as the chain reaction was alternately initiated by the attainment of a critical geometry and then quenched as radiolytic gas bubbles modified this geometry. Under these circumstances pulse duration is thought to have been of the order of 100 ms with intervals of several seconds between pulses (ORNL 1958). Because of a long time constant and high sensitivity the radiation monitor in an adjacent building did not register clearly the fine structure of the radiation pulses. There can therefore be no incontrovertible proof of the precise sequence and relative intensities of the pulses. However laboratory experiments indicate that the first pulse can be considerably larger than subsequent pulses (Lecorch and Seale 1973). This is because, in the absence of a raised ambient neutron fluence, the conditions required for criticality can be exceeded by a considerable margin and only when a sufficiently large statistical fluctuation in the ambient neutron fluence arises will criticality occur. Subsequent pulses are triggered as soon as criticality is achieved by the now raised neutron fluence. The observations, by two of the exposed, of a 'blue flash' immediately prior to the alarm sounding (ORNL 1958), but not a second flash after the alarm sounded, would be consistent with Cerenkov radiation resulting from the first large pulse of radiation.

Given then that exposure at Y12 is likely to have been principally from one aspect it might seem reasonable to base dose estimates on the liberal amount of information provided to the inquiry by those present (ORNL 1958). Apart from the fact that persons having undergone a traumatic event are not always reliable witnesses, there are good reasons for being sceptical of the evidence in this particular case. Immediately following the accident there were two available methods for making preliminary dose estimates while the results of the dosimetry from the sodium activation measurements were awaited. These were a) deductions from the indium foil badges and b) calculations based upon the total number of fissions thought to have occurred in the drum ($\sim 10^{18}$) and the positions of the exposed individuals (see table 1). The results obtained by the first method (indium foil activation measurements) agree tolerably well with the FCD's for neutrons ultimately determined from the sodium-24 measurements but the calculations based on positions of individuals at the time of exposure all overestimate the dose. This is probably due to the exposed individual receiving only a fraction of the total fission yield, (it was estimated that 10^{17} fissions occurred in the first pulse) but the dose calculated for individual A (ORNL 1958) represented a far greater over-estimate than for any of the other exposed individuals. This calculation was based upon his claim to have been six feet from the drum when the accident occurred. The lack of agreement between physical measurements (of the indium foils and of sodium-24 in blood) and calculations based on personal recollections summarised in table 1 must cast doubt on the accuracy of those recollections. In view of this there must be considerable uncertainty in the doses received by individuals exposed at Y12. To reflect this uncertainty in the dosimetric reassessment based on the Cross (1981) model, the tissue kerma for neutrons was determined assuming exposure from the front or back (the maximum value for the ratio A/V) and from the side (the minimum value for A/V) these resulting in the minimum and maximum estimates of tissue kerma to which the individual might have been exposed respectively (Baverstock and Ash 1983).

At Vinca, exposure lasted several minutes and accounts of the movements of the individuals during the exposure period are unclear. Since over such an extended period some movement was likely it seems more reasonable in this case to assume that an average geometry might apply. This is however only an assumption and as such is also uncertain.

In 1974 an international intercomparison experiment on dosimetry of the Vinca neutron spectrum was held at Vinca (Miric 1977). From the results reported, estimates of the errors involved in measurements on these neutrons can be made and these were used as the basis for expressing the uncertainty in the reassessed doses for individuals at Vinca. Uncertainty due to factors such as orientation are not included since they are unquantifiable.

Tissue kerma for gamma-rays can be determined from the ratios of first collision doses measured at the calibration experiments (ORNL 1958

TABLE 1

Summary of first collision doses for neutrons at Y12

| Individual | First collision dose for neutrons (cGy) Based upon:- | | | activation of ^{24}Na in blood | |
	reported positions and total yield of 10^{18} fissions*	reported positions and first pulse cf 10^{17} fissions	activation of indium foils*	at time of accident*	present estimates+
A	4899	490	48	96	73-143
B	770	77	31	71	54-106
C	628	63	50	81	68-133
D	735	74	40	86	65-128
E	397	40	56	62	46-91
F	204	20	14.7	18	14-27

* ORNL (1958)
+ Baverstock and Ash (1983)

and IAEA 1961). From the tissue kerma for neutrons and gamma-rays it is possible to obtain tissue doses in bone marrow with the help of a model for calculating bone marrow dose based on measured bone marrow distributions in cadavers (Jones 1977). The neutron component of dose can be divided into two sub-components, namely the charged particle dose (high LET in character and therefore requiring modification by a value for RBE) and the auto-gamma dose. As mentioned above, auto-gamma dose is important mainly in connection with low energy neutrons which give rise to relatively little charged particle dose but which are as effective at producing auto-gamma rays as are higher energy neutrons when they are captured. In fact, because of their limited penetrating ability, the low energy neutrons in the Vinca spectrum were absorbed mainly in superficial tissues.

The RBE chosen to allow for the extra effectiveness of the charged particle component of the neutron dose is 3. This is based on experiments on hamster cells irradiated in vitro with neutrons of various energies and applies to survival levels in the region of 10% (Kellerer et al 1976). There is bound to be uncertainty in this figure since the circumstances in which the value of 3 was determined are very different from those applying to bone marrow in man and shielded by several centimetres of other tissue. However, experiments in goats by Edmondson and Batchelor (1971) indicate that an RBE for neutrons based on exposure rather than tissue dose would be about 0.8. In terms of charged particle dose within the bone marrow allowing for attenuation in more superficial tissues, these experiments suggest an RBE of about 3 would be appropriate assuming that the marrow is uniformly irradiated.

The auto-gamma dose can be computed for the appropriate neutron spectrum from the tables given by Jones (1977), and the dose to bone marrow from the external gamma irradiation can be computed by allowing for the attenuation in the superficial tissues.

The low LET equivalent doses for neutrons and gamma-rays as computed by this technique are given in table 2 as ranges; the lower and upper limits based on the two possible extremes of orientation with respect to the radiation source for the Y12 accident and on errors estimated from the intercomparison experiments (Mirić 1977) for Vinca.

TABLE 2

Bone marrow doses and indicators of severity of effect for individuals exposed at Y12 and Vinca

Accident	Individuals	Equivalent low LET dose ranges in cGy for + :-						Severity of 2nd phase symptoms at between 20 and 35 days ‡	Integrated blood count score* at days		
		Neutrons		γ-rays		Total			30	60	120
		lower	upper	lower	upper	lower	upper				
Y12	A	91	143	171	296	263	439	+	43	61	61
	B	68	106	127	219	195	325	−	29	46	46
	C	85	133	160	276	245	409	+	36	55	55
	D	82	128	154	266	236	394	+	21	32	32
	E	58	91	110	189	168	280	−	23	39	39
	F	17	27	33	56	50	83	−	5	5	5
	G	17	27	33	56	50	83	−	0	0	0
	H	6	9	10	18	16	27	−	0	0	0
Vinca	H	37	51	133	181	170	230	+++	29	56	62
	V	51	69	181	245	232	314	Died	77	−	−
	G	49	67	134	182	184	250	+++	46	57	63
	M	49	67	178	240	227	307	+++	71	88	92
	D	50	68	134	182	184	250	+++	66	114	127
	B	25	35	83	111	108	146	+	20	28	35

+ Taken from Baverstock and Ash (1983)

‡ Increasing severity denoted by number of plus signs

* Taken from Wald and Thoma (1961) and comprises the scores after 30, 60 and 120 days post exposure for neutrophils, lymphocytes and platelets only

Symptomatology and treatment

The symptoms suffered by the exposed individuals at Y12, especially in the latter phases of radiation sickness at between 20 and 30 days post exposure, were considerably milder than those experienced by the individuals exposed at Vinca (table 2). This qualitative conclusion is supported by the results of Wald and Thoma (1962) who attempted to quantify the damage to bone marrow by "scoring" the departure from normality for several cell types in blood following the exposure. Their results show significantly higher scores for those exposed at Vinca than for those exposed at Y12; this applies from the earliest times and certainly before the treatment given to the Vinca cases is likely to have influenced the scoring. The relationship of these scores to the low LET equivalent doses to bone marrow is also shown in table 2. Clearly there is very little correlation between the blood count score and the dose for the two accidents although within a single accident there seems to be a reasonable correlation.

The symptoms of bleeding, fever etc. between 20 and 40 days post-exposure for those exposed at Vinca are all typical of severe bone marrow depression and the pattern of bone marrow changes is qualitatively similar for both accidents. However, at Vinca there is the suggestion, particularly in subject V who died, of some gastro-intestinal involvement. The cause of death for individual V was intestinal obstruction but this was at 32 days post exposure which is atypically late for gut syndrome alone which occurs usually within a week or two of exposure. There must therefore be doubt as to the relevance of V's death to the question of bone marrow syndrome in man but there can be little doubt that the bone marrow in the most heavily exposed individuals at Vinca was severely damaged.

Discussion

The lack of agreement between dose and symptomatology at the two accidents must limit their value as sources of information relevant to man's sensitivity to the effects of uniform, whole-body irradiation unless some explanation for the difference can be found. The dosimetries for the two accidents have been put on a comparable basis and as much account as is feasible has been taken of the uncertainties in individual doses. It would seem, therefore, more profitable to examine the other differences between the two accidents for a possible explanation. These lie principally in the duration of exposure and in the quality of the radiations involved. We then have to determine whether, as a result of one or other of these factors, the doses at Y12 are unrepresentatively high or those at Vinca are unrepresentatively low. The choice seems to lie in the following two explanations:-

a) at Y12 the greater part of the dose was received in such a short time interval that exposure was essentially from one aspect only and that therefore some marrow deposits were significantly protected from damage by the shielding provided by the remainder of the body; or alternatively;

b) that at Vinca the 'softness' of the neutron radiation led to excessive irradiation of tissues other than bone marrow (in particular the gastro-intestinal tract) and this resulted in the severe symptomatology observed at Vinca.

It should be noted that these two explanations are not mutually exclusive: the acceptance of one does not imply anything regarding the validity of the other.

On the basis of the physical circumstances of the Y12 accident explanation a) seems quite feasible. The radiation was emitted in pulses, the first one being of about 100 milliseconds duration and releasing the energy from about 10^{17} fissions or about 10% of the overall release (ORNL 1958). The reported blue flash, consistent with Cerenkov radiation, supports the concept of a brief but very high energy pulse. It could be postulated that during the time it took the employees to walk from the building on hearing the alarm, they were exposed to a second pulse of radiation thus making their exposure more homogeneous. It is, of course, not possible to rule out entirely this possibility, however, if this was the case a curious anomaly has to be explained, namely why the doses to individuals C and E are not nearly identical, since these two workers are alleged to have left the scene of the accident together (ORNL 1958). In fact the sodium-24 activities measured in C and E are more or less consistent with the ratio of distances from the drum at which they were alleged to have been. It therefore seems probable that if there was a second pulse which resulted in irradiation of those leaving the building it was only of minor consequence to the dose.

The neutron energy spectrum at Vinca was soft because of the moderating effect of the D_2O on neutrons generated in the core of the reactor. Most of the neutrons that escaped the reactor were of very low energy and as such had very little penetrability. The result is that the energy spectrum for neutrons at the depth in tissue appropriate for bone marrow or for GI tract (as opposed to that free in air) is similar to the spectrum at Yl2. Thus, from the neutron component at least, only the most superficial tissues of those exposed at Vinca, namely skin, is likely to have received a significantly greater dose for a given FCD when compared with those exposed at Yl2. In fact erythema of the skin was noted at Vinca but not for Yl2.

Little seems to have been reported of the energy distribution for gamma-rays at Vinca. Apart from the prompt gamma-rays generated during the fission reaction, there will have been a contribution from delayed gamma-rays from fission products and auto gamma-rays from the capture of neutrons by hydrogen contaminating the D_2O and by ^{238}U. Further there will have been activation gamma-rays from the interaction of the neutrons with all the surrounding materials including the aluminium containment of the reactor itself. Estimates made at the time suggest that prompt gamma-rays predominated (IAEA 1962). Since these were subject to absorption by the D_2O and fuel rods the spectrum will have been 'softer' than a fission spectrum. However, this would also be the case to some extent at Yl2 where the gamma-rays emanated from a uranium containing solution. The extent to which the gamma spectrum at Vinca was different from that at Yl2 is therefore a matter for speculation. What maybe important however is that the source of radiation at Vinca was larger than that at Yl2 and that those exposed were considerably closer to the source and in an environment with nearby walls, in which scattering would be important. These features would tend to increase the uniformity of dose distribution in the exposed individuals.

On balance, therefore, it seems reasonable to assume that it is more likely that the Yl2 victims' symptoms were unrepresentatively mild for the doses they received due to non-uniform irradiation. As was stated earlier, this does not imply that the doses and symptomatology received at Vinca are typical of the effects on man, and there remains uncertainty concerning the nature of the death of subject V.

Two other sources of data come to mind in connection with the sensitivity of man to radiation-induced bone marrow failure. These are a) the experience from the Japanese bombings in Hiroshima and Nagasaki and b) patients treated with radiotherapy.

There are a number of reasons why the Japanese experience may not be typical of a normally healthy population exposed to radiation alone. There is evidence that the population was undernourished at the time of the bombings but more importantly there is the possibility that the radiation injury was compounded by the effects of heat and blast. This is because with bombs the size of those employed in Japan the area of more or less lethal radiation damage approximates closely to that for lethal heat and blast damage (SIPRI 1983). It might, therefore, be expected that if deaths following within 60 days of the bombings were attributed solely to the effects of radiation, the doses causing such deaths may well be somewhat smaller than the doses required in the absence of other injuries.

Patients treated with radiotherapy also present problems since they can hardly be described as normally healthy. However, at least one particular group, namely patients suffering from Ewing's sarcoma, who were treated in Canada with total body irradiation to control disseminated disease, provide a potentially useful population. Briefly, 20 patients (mainly teenagers) were treated to 3 Gy low LET irradiation to the mid-line of the body in a period of about 20 minutes. The dose was more or less uniform since the patients were turned over half way through the irradiation. Among these 20 patients there were no deaths within 60 days of exposure (Rider and Hasselback 1968).

The Ewings sarcoma patients appear to be the best human evidence available and would suggest that mortality among normally healthy persons exposed briefly to 3 Gy low LET ionising radiation probably does not exceed a few per cent. This conclusion does not appear to agree well with the experience from Vinca although the uncertainties are great enough to allow an accommodation especially if the dose response for man is steep.

CONCLUSION

It must therefore be concluded that the basis of our knowledge of man's sensitivity to the effects of brief whole-body exposure to low LET radiation is tenuous indeed. The relatively few accidents that have occurred as the result of man's exploitation of radiation have not contributed greatly to our knowledge, largely because of the difficulty of accurately and reliably reconstructing the event in order to make dosimetric estimates. This problem is the more critical since it is likely that man, in common with other animals, will exhibit a steep dose response curve, the dose for very high percentage mortalities in a population being about twice that for low percentage mortalities (Baverstock et al unpublished results).

REFERENCES

BAVERSTOCK K.F. and ASH P.J.N.D., 1983. A review of radiation accidents involving whole body exposure and the relevance to the $LD_{50/60}$ for man. Brit.J.Radiol 56, 837

CROSS, W.G., 1981. Neutron activation of sodium in phantoms and the human body. *Health Physics*, 41, 105-121.

DELAFIELD, H.J., DENNIS, J.A. and GIBSON, J.A.B., 1973. Nuclear accident dosimetry, Pt III: Interpretation and data. AERE R7487.

HURST, G.S., RITCHIE, R.H. and EMERSON, L.C., 1959. Accidental radiation excursion at the Oak Ridge Y12 plant. III. Determination of radiation doses. *Health Physics*, 2, 121-133.

HURST, G.S., RITCHIE, R.H., SANDERS, F.W., REINHARDT, T.W., AUXIER, J.A., WAGNER, E.B., CALLIHAN, A.D. and MORGAN, K.Z., 1961. Dosimetry investigation of the Yugoslav accident. *Health Physics*, 5, 179-202.

I.A.E.A., 1962. The Vinca dosimetry experiment. Technical Report Series No. 6. (International Atomic Energy Agency, Vienna).

JONES, T.D., 1977. CHORD operators for cell survival models and insult assessment to active bone marrow. *Radiation Research*, 71, 269-283.

LECORCHE, P. and SEALE, R.L., 1973. Review of the experiments performed to determine the radiological consequences of a criticality accident. Report no. Y-CDC-12.

MIRIC, I., 1977. Nuclear accident dosimetry. Report of the 3rd IAEA intercomparison experiment at Vinca, Yugoslavia. Report MG-140.

O.R.N.L., 1958. Accidental radiation excursion at the Y12 plant. Final Report Y 1234. (Oak Ridge National Laboratory, Oak Ridge, Tennessee).

RIDER, W.D. and HASSELBACK, R., 1968. The symptomatic and haematological disturbance following total body irradiation of 300 rad gamma-ray irradiation. In Guidelines to radiological health, Public Health Service Publication, no. 999-RH-33, pp. 139-144 (U.S. Department of Health Education and Welfare, Washington D.C.).

SIPRI, 1981. Nuclear radiation in warfare, p.70. (Taylor and Francis, London).

WALD, N. and THOMA, G.F., 1961. Radiation accidents: medical aspects of neutron and gamma-ray exposures. Oak Ridge National Laboratory Report, ORNL 2748, Part B.

TOTAL BODY IRRADIATION AND LD 50 IN MAN

ANN BARRETT

The Royal Marsden Hospital, Radiotherapy Department,
Downs Road, Sutton, Surrey SM2 5PT United Kingdom.

Estimates of the dose of whole body irradiation in man which would be expected to kill half the exposed population (the LD_{50}) have varied considerably. There has been a tendency for more recent estimates to give higher doses which reflects recognition of measures which may influence the outcome of such an exposure. Thus Warren and Bowers (1950) suggested an LD_{50} of 3 Gy, Mole (1975) a higher value of 4.5 Gy and two other groups more than 5 Gy (US NRC reactor safety study, 1975, Deutsche Risikostudie Kernkraftwerke, 1980).

Perhaps of more interest in man would be the ability to predict the likelihood of recovery for any given dose. From animal studies, it has been deduced that almost all animals receiving 1.3 times the LD_{50} dose will die and that no deaths will occur when doses of less than half this value are received (Jones 1981). Other workers have suggested a threshold for man of 2 Gy below which no deaths will occur after whole body irradiation. There is probably an inherent error of ±10% in estimating LD_{50} doses and species variability must be considered, although the slope of the curve relating dose to mortality is probably similar from species to species.

The LD_{50} in man is related to death from bone marrow damage. If this can be avoided, as for example by bone marrow transplantation, other organ tolerances may be critical. Data from upper half body treatments suggests that with high dose rate (3 to 4 Gy/min) irradiation, doses of 10 Gy will produce pneumonitis in up to 80% of patients, many of whom will die of this complication (Van Dijk et al, 1981). Similarly, in patients receiving 10 Gy whole body irradiation before bone marrow transplantation, there is a 30% incidence of pneumonitis with a 15% mortality occurring within 100 days after irradiation (Thomas et al, 1977). Although the aetiology is multifactorial, death from radiation lung damage can be predicted after doses of more than 12 Gy.

In transplanted patients, the gut syndrome is not an important cause of morbidity. Its lethality in accident victims is perhaps related to its association with marrow suppression and infection which are prevented with transplantation.

The lethal dose for therapeutic irradiation can therefore be defined in terms of bone marrow toxicity in untransplanted patients or lung toxicity in transplanted patients.

Data for calculating LD_{50} doses in man are derived from three sources; treatment with low LET radiation of patients who usually are suffering from malignant disease; from criticality accidents; and from other accidental exposures to whole body irradiation.

In 1963, before effective drugs were available to treat Ewings sarcoma, a rare bone tumour in children, whole body irradiation was used to try to eliminate micrometastatic disease. Doses of 0.5 to 2.2 Gy were reported to give no side effects, although there were transient falls in white cell and platelet counts. At 3 to 4 Gy, bone marrow depression was seen and necessitated hospital admission and support with antibiotics and blood products for up to two months. Only one patient out of 26 treated died and this was related to complications other than those directly attributable to radiation (Rider and Hasselbach, 1968).

From a group of patients with advanced cancer treated with whole body doses of 3±0.3 Gy reported by Lusbaugh et al (1967), an estimated LD_{50} of 2.8±0.4 Gy was suggested but their poor general condition will undoubtably contribute to this.

Data derived from criticality and several other radiation accidents are well summarized by Smith in the NRPB report R139 (1983) where he has drawn up a normal probability dose-mortality curve for man. Interpretation of data from accidents is difficult since in many cases exposure is not uniform or accurate dosimetry was not available. In the Oak Ridge (Y-12) accident, estimated doses were either in the range 1.7 to 2.6 Gy assuming an antero-posterior exposure or 2.8 to 4.4 Gy assuming a lateral one. All seven exposed workers survived.

Some accidental exposures have given information about protracted irradiation which confirms animal experimental data suggesting an increase in LD_{50} doses as exposure times are increased for the same dose (Corp and Neal, 1959).

Many factors which modify the LD_{50} in man must be considered. These may be classified as:
     - radiation related
     - inherent patient characteristics
     - external modifications

Radiation associated factors to be considered when stating an LD_{50} for man include, as well as the total dose, the dose rate or time over which the irradiation is received, the type of irradiation, which will often be mixed neutron and gamma in accident situations, the volume of tissue irradiated and considerations of beam direction.

Age, sex and general health status may affect the LD_{50}. In the context of bone marrow transplantation, whole body irradiation is increasingly poorly tolerated as patients' age increases. Some reports have suggested an increased incidence of radiation side effects such as vomiting occurring at lower doses in women which may reflect a generalized increased sensitivity. Any chronic illness present at the time of exposure is likely to contribute to increased mortality.

External modifications may be of most significance in suggesting revised LD_{50} levels. Recovery is known to have occurred in three individuals after exposure to single therapeutic whole body doses of 10 Gy when initial bone marrow or foetal liver grafts failed with subsequent autologous reconstitution. Some animal experimental data has shown that rabbits can survive much higher doses of whole body irradiation if a temporary graft can be achieved (Speck et al, 1975).

It is not known what proportion of haemopoeitic stem cells remain after 10 Gy whole body dose or how many stem cells are needed to repopulate the marrow after such treatment. A cell load of $2x10^8$ per kg is given during a bone marrow transplant which has been estimated to be about 1/100 of the normal marrow content.

Periods of complete aplasia of up to six weeks can be managed by isolation techniques with sterile precautions, gut decontamination, use of intra-venous antibiotics and support with blood and platelet transfusions. Beyond this time, infection with opportunistic organisms and fungi becomes increasingly likely leading to a fatal outcome.

For people exposed to whole body doses greater than the established LD_{50}, protective isolation with the supportive measures outlined above may raise this value by 10-20%.

The association of radiation damage with other types of injury (burns, fractures, etc.) will increase the risk of bleeding and infection and death may be expected with lower total whole body doses. Radiation induced aplasia may also impair repair processes leading to a higher complication rate and mortality from conventional injuries.

Thus, in man it seems of limited usefulness to describe one LD_{50} value. The factors mentioned above should be considered and values qualified as LD_{50} with maximal supportive care (?5-6 Gy) or LD_{50} with associated severe injury (LD_{50}?2 Gy).

208

References:

Corp, M. and Neal, F.E., 1959. The modification of acute mortality in mice by variation of the dose-rate and the overall time of radiation. Int.J.Radiat.Biol., 1, 256.

Deutsche Risikostudie Kernkraftwerke, 1980. Eine Untersuchung zu den durch Storfalle in Kernkraftwerken verursachten Risiko, Verlag, TUV, Rheinland.

Dijk, J. van, Keane, T., Kan, S., Rider, W.D., and Fryer, C.J.H., 1981. Radiation pneumonitis following large single dose irradiation: A re-evaluation based on absolute dose to lung. Int.J.Radiat.Oncol.Biol. Phys. 7, 461.

Jones, T.D., 1981. Hematologic syndrome in man modelled from mammalian lethality. Health Phys., 41, 83.

Lusbaugh, C.C., Comas, F. and Hofstra, R., 1967. Clinical studies on the radiation effects in man. Radiat. Res., suppl. 7, 398.

Mole, R.H., 1975. Deductions about survival curve parameters from iso-effect radiation regimes: observations on lethality after whole body irradiation of mice. In: Cell survival after low doses of radiation (Alper, T, ed), Proceedings 6th L.H.Gray Conference Chicester, Wiley, p. 229.

Rider, W.D. and Hasselbach, R., 1968. The symptomatic and haematological disturbance following total body irradiation of 300 rad gamma ray condition. Guidelines to radiological health. Washington DC, US Department of Health, Education and Welfare, p. 139.

Smith, H., 1983. Dose-effect relationships for early response to total body irradiation. National Radiological Protection Board-R 139.

Speck, B., Buckner, C.D., Jeannet, M. et al, 1975. Erfahrungen mit der allogenen und isogenen Knockenmarktransplantation bei aplastischer Anamie und akuter Leukaemia. Schweiz Med. Wochenstr. 105 (47) 1574.

Thomas, E.D., Buckner, C.D. et al, 1977. One hundred patients with acute leukaemia treated by chemotherapy, total body irradiation and allogenic marrow transplantation. Blood, 49, 511.

US NRC, 1975. An assessment of accident risks in US commercial nuclear power plants. US Nuclear Regulatory Commission, WASH-1400, appendix F.

Warren, S. and Bowers, J.Z., 1950. The acute radiation syndrome in man. Ann.Int.Med., 32, 207.

BIOLOGICAL FACTORS AFFECTING THE OCCURRENCE OF RADIATION SYNDROMES

T.M. FLIEDNER, W. NOTHDURFT AND H. HEIT
Department of Clinical Physiology and Occupational Medicine, University of
Ulm, D-7900 Ulm/Donau, Fed. Rep. of Germany

1. Introduction

The effects of increasing doses of ionizing radiation on the survival time
of a variety of mammalian species have been reviewed previously (1). From
the data obtained, 3 parts of the "survival curves" may be distinguished
which are related to the radiation effects on "critical" organ systems.
Up to a total dose of 1000 cGy, there is a dose dependent reduction in the
survival times of exposed animals until a plateau is achieved at about
3 - 4 days for several conventionally bread animals, such as the mouse,
rat, dog, swine and goat. Death in this first dose dependent part of the
survival curve is due to the failure of hemopoiesis to supply sufficient
numbers of mature blood cells, causing the so-called "hemopoietic syndrome".
The second part of the survival curve is characterized by a plateau with
respect to survival times of exposed animals that extend from about 1000
cGy to 5000 or even 10 000 cGy, depending on the species. The animal species mentioned die 3 - 4 days after exposure independent of the dose
given. The level of the plateau is, however, at about 6 - 7 days for species such as germfree mice, guinea pigs, but also monkeys. Pathophysiological studies indicate, that the survival time of 3 - 4 and 6 - 7 days
respectively in these animal species is primarily determined by the fact,
that these doses between 1000 and 5000 or even 10 000 cGy destroy the
stem-cell population of the intestinal tract and thereby cause a subsequent denudation of the intestinal mucosa resulting in a severe disturbance
of the electrolyte balance with fluid loss and microbial invasion. Since
at such radiation dose levels the bone marrow function is destroyed as
well, granulocytopenia is produced which - together with the denudation
of the intestinal surface - results in a "gastrointestinal syndrome",
characterized by diarrhoea and bacterial infections. The third part of
the survival curve is again dose dependent. The higher the dose beyond
5000 or 10 000 cGy, the shorter is the survival time. If the death is
within minutes of exposure, one may call it "death under the beam". This
is due to a severe perturbation of the central nervous regulation and co-
ordination of organ functions.

It is the purpose of this presentation to examine means and ways by which
the dose - (life expectancy)effect-relationship described may be modified
by biological factors. How far is it possible to influence this typical
dose-response pattern by affecting the hemopoietic and/or the gastrointestinal syndrome by suitable therapeutic regimens?

2. Modification of the Gastrointestinal Syndrome by Specific Supportive Care Measures

It was indicated above that the survival time of germfree mice at dose levels between 1000 and 5000 cGy is about 6-7 days in comparison to conventionally maintained mice that survive such lethal exposures for only about 3 - 4 days. This obvious higher resistance of germfree mice is also reflected in a higher value for LD 50/5 days (i.e. the dose which kills 50 % of the exposed animals within 5 days), which is 2000 cGy in comparison to 1260 cGy for conventional mice (1). A lot of experimental work was performed elucidating the mechanism of this observations. It was found that the generation time of crypt cells in germfree mice and the migration transit times of villus cells is about twice as long than in normal mice (2).

Furthermore, the time for the denudation of the intestinal epithelium of germfree mice is about twice as long as in normal mice. Hence, the occurrence of the gastrointestinal syndrome is remarkably delayed under germfree conditions. It was also observed that, in parallel to the LD 50/5 days, the LD 50/30 days, i.e. the LD 50 for the bone marrow syndrome, is different between conventional and germfree mice: v.d. Waaij (3) determined the values with 610 cGy and 840 cGy respectively.

From these studies it became obvious, that there are biological factors that change the occurence of the radiation syndromes. In summary, the "gastrointestinal syndrome" can be modified by mainly two factors, supply of sufficient fluids and control of pathogenic microorganisms. It was shown by Taketa (4) that a total body exposure of rats results in a 100 % lethality within 6 days if no support is given. However, there is zero percent mortality within 6 days if the animals are treated with a combination of antibiotics and balanced salt solutions.

These basic observations have been confirmed time and again in preclinical studies in dogs but more recently also in man. In bone marrow transplantation studies in dogs, monkeys and man there is now sufficient evidence to show that exposed individuals can survive the first 10 days after a "supralethal" exposure in the dose range from 800 to 1500 cGy (that is after doses between 2 and 3 times the "LD 50/30 or 60 days") if supportive care is administered. In our hands it is important to administer to dogs given total body irradiation at dose levels of 1000 - 2000 cGy electrolyte solutions in an amount of up to 2000 ml per day in order to combat the fluid loss caused by the "gastrointestinal syndrome". Maybe this fluid replacement therapy can best be compared to the schedule of burn treatments which is based on the fraction of injured skin. In the case or radiation exposure - one may visualize the biological consequences of a denuded intestinal surface as an "internal burn damage", requiring a fierce and continuous fluid replacement determined by the fluid loss from the denuded gastrointestinal surfaces. However, in all these species mentioned, such "supralethal" doses of irradiation produce a profound granulocytopenia (3 - 4 days in dogs after 1200 cGy, 4 - 5 days in man after 1000 or more cGy) at the same time the intestinal denudation takes place. Thus, the pathogenetic microorganisms of the intestinal flora will find no competent biological barrier and will overwhelm the irradiated organism. This fact has lead to the concept that two possibilities exist alone or in combination to prevent death from bacterial infection as one element of the pathogenesis of the gastrointestinal syndrome. The first possibility is the administration of suitable antibiotics. The systematic administration of systemic antibiotics in dogs - first introduced by E.D. Thomas (5) - is still used in bone marrow transplantation studies to overcome early lethality by bacterial infections. We are usually using a combination of penicilline and the amino-glucoside netilmycine. However, in clinical circumstances, new approaches are being used based on extensive animal experimentation. These consist mainly of a "microbial decontamination" of the individual to be exposed to an otherwise lethal dose of irradiation by means of non-resorbable antibiotics. In mice, it was found that a systematic oral administration of a combination of neomycin, bacitracin and carbenicillium results in a complete removal of all bacteria from the intestinal tract and consequently from the skin if the animals are placed into a germfree environment (sterile cage, fed with sterile food) (6). In human beings, a similar approach is feasible. One can remove a large component of the microbial flora by antibiotic therapy and maintain such a "gnotobiotic state" in a germfree isolation system. In our transplant team at Ulm University, a specially designed germfree isolation system made from plastic material is used for treating leukemic patients with total body irradiation and subsequent bone marrow transplantation (7).

It should be mentioned that the microbial infection caused by the gastrointestinal syndrome and by granulocytopenia as a consequence of "supralethal" whole body radiation exposure has also been successfully modified by transfusion of large quantities of granulocytes. An early example of this approach was the treatment of pseudomonas infection of leukemic patients by leukocyte transfusions (8).

Thus, it is concluded that it is quite possible to alter the radiation induced gastrointestinal syndrome and reduce or eliminate lethal consequences in all mammalian species studied so far. In mice, rats, dogs, monkeys and man, early mortality (3 - 6 days after exposure) at dose levels in excess of two to four times the LD 50/30 or 60 days can be reduced to zero if supportive care is employed. This must include a carefully balanced fluid replacement to make up for any excess fluid loss caused by the consequences of damage to the intestinal surface. It must also include a regimen to prevent the uncontrolled growth and invasion of the organism by its own endogenous intestinal microbial flora. This can be achieved by administration of suitable antibiotics or - more recently developed - by performing a "selective decontamination" removing the pathogeneic or potentially pathogeneic organisms and leaving the anaerobic flora intact. In case of a "complete" decontamination by trying to eliminate the entire microbial flora and producing a "germfree state" even in human beings (9), the antibiotic treatment has to be combined with the maintenance of the organism within a sterile environment ("life island", Ulm isolation system) for the period of lowered resistence of the body against microbial invasion. Such a therapeutic potentiality may have to be supplemented by granulocyte transfusions in order to eliminate pathogenic microorganisms from "niches" that may not be reached even by extensive antibiotic therapy. Granulocyte transfusions do not present technical problems since equipment became available to perform leukocytaphereses in human donors.

3. Modification of the Hemopoietic Syndrome by Specific Supportive Care Measures

In experimental animals as well as in human beings exposure to ionizing radiation in the dose range of the LD 50/30 or 60 days, respectively, is followed by a "hemopoietic syndrome". It has been shown that up to three cell systems are involved in radiation induced lethality at this dose level. Which cell systems contribute most to this lethality depends on the species. From Fig. 1 it can be seen, that in the rat lethality is

Fig.1:

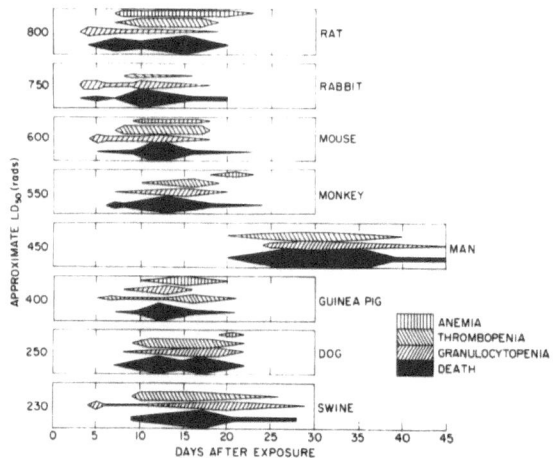

correlated with anemia and thrombocytopenia, whereas the granulocyte system is not involved. In the dog, anemia is no problem, but the animal may die from the consequences of granulocytopenia and thrombopenia. In human beings, there is - at this dose level - no significant contribution to lethality from anemia. However, granulocytopenia and thrombopenia are of importance. The time sequence of events is quite different in human beings due to the particular cell turnover kinetics in comparison to other species.

The dose-effect relationship in all species examined at the LD 50/30 or 60 day level can certainly be modified extensively, if the consequences of the anemia, the granulocytopenia or the thrombocytopenia are treated by supportive care or replacement therapy in a systematic and pathogenetically justified manner. Thus, in the rat, red cell replacement and platelet-transfusions combined with antibiotics, if necessary, for manifested infections will allow the animal to survive a radiation exposure at the level of a LD 50/30 day. In the dog, platelet transfusions combined with a systemic and systemic antibiotic therapy will overcome the critical period of hemopoietic failure which is apparent between the 10th and 20th day after exposure to an LD 50 for the bone marrow syndrome. The effectiveness of such an approach has been demonstrated by Sorensen et al. in 1960 (10). In human beings, the same principles are being employed. In this case, the extensive knowledge about the time sequence of cellular

events after a "mid-lethal" whole body exposure, characterized by granulocytopenia and thrombopenia in the 4th and 5th week after exposure
allows one to combat the expected consequences. The infections can be prevented or treated by antibiotic therapy which may be prophylactic if
gnotobiotic environment technics are being employed. More recently, the
advent of the concepts of "selective decontamination" (as proposed by
the "European Gnotobiotic Project Group" (11)) may well allow such a
treatment on the open ward. If necessary, such an antibacterial treatment may have to be supplemented by granulocyte transfusion. Bleeding
due to thrombopenia can be prevented by administering blood platelets
when thrombopenia becomes extensive (i.e. when the platelet level falls
markedly below 50 000 per mm³ blood).

In conclusion, radiation exposures at the dose level of an LD 50/30 days
or 60 days, respectively,will not result in any lethality if the hematological consequences are specifically dealt with. These consequences
differ between the species under consideration. If anemia is a major
factor contributing to lethality, then red cell replacement will correct
this deficiency until autochthonous hemopoietic regeneration takes a
hold. If granulocytopenia and hence bacterial infection contribute to
lethality, then gnotobiotic approaches have to be used such as complete
antibiotic decontamination and maintenance of the gnotobiotic state in a
germfree environment or "selective" decontamination until the granulocyte concentration in the blood is again well above 1000/mm³ due to hemopoietic regeneration. It may also be necessary to add granulocyte transfusions to the therapeutic regimen to overcome infections through a re-
sistent microbial flora. If thrombocytopenic bleeding is the major cause
for radiation induced lethality, then platelet transfusions must be
applied.

The supportive care and replacement therapy is certainly able to modify
extensively the severeness of the hemopoietic radiation syndrome and
may well overcome its lethal consequences. This concept and its practical
application is of course based on the assumption that the damage to
the cell renewal systems (gastrointestinal epithelium and - in particular -
the hemopoietic tissue) is reversible and not irreversible. In other words,
the surviving fractions of the stem cell populations must be capable of
a spontaneous regeneration without external help.

4. Modification of the Radiation Syndromes by Stem-Cell Substitution

The possibilities of modifying the radiation syndromes by replacement
(electrolytes, blood cells) and administration of antibiotics find their
limitations in a decisive problem. The question is always, whether or
not a sufficient number of uninjured stem-cells have survived from which
a spontaneous recovery of blood cell production may take place.

As far as the intestinal epithelium is concerned, it is well known that
after a total body exposure a spontaneous regeneration is possible even
after a dose in the range of 2000 - 3000 cGy when given as one fraction.
This is a reflection of the relatively low radiation sensitivity of the
crypt stem cell population. In general it is fair to say that an irreversible damage of the intestinal epithelium will be observed only at
dose levels that are high enough to cause death by other means (cardio-
vascular or central nervous damage).

The <u>central nervous</u> system syndrome is the consequence of the effect of ionizing radiation on those organ systems that are required to coordinate body functions and include not only radiation effects on the neurons themselves but much more on the supporting tissue. Thus, the symptomes are related with the effect of radiation on the vascular system causing edema in confined spaces.

The situation is quite different from the <u>hemopoietic tissue</u>. It is well known that the hemopoietic stem cell population is characterized by an extensive radiation sensitivity. Depending on the system (species) investigated and the methods used by different authors, the D_o for pluripotent hemopoietic bone marrow stem cells is in the order of 95 cGy and 105 cGy (12). This means, that a total body irradiation of the mouse with a dose in the range of the LD 50/30 days i. e. approximately 700 cGy reduces the size of the stem cell pool to such an extend that only one out of 1000 stem cells remains from which a spontaneous regeneration of the stem cell pool can be expected to occur. Therefore, after irradiation the critical question is related to the estimation of the size of the stem cell pool from which a regeneration may commence. From consideration of Morley et al. (13) one may assume, that a reduction of the stem cell pool to less than 2 % of its original size may be the critical threshold. If this value is reached or exceeded, then the marrow seems to be injured to such an extend that a spontaneous recovery cannot be expected in a reasonable period of time.

It is in this situation - well reviewed previously (1) - that the use of a "substitution therapy", supplemented by a carefully administered supportive care to overcome the consequences of transient intestinal and/or hemopoietic failure, can modify drastically the dose-effect-curve of whole body exposure of untreated individuals.

Substitution therapy in this sense means the goal to substitute the stem cells lost by radiation with stem cells of unlimited potentialities of replication and differentiation. This field of research was opened by Lorenz, Uphoff, Reid and Shelton in 1951 (14) who were able to show that bone marrow cell transfusions can overcome hemopoietic death by initiating a speedy recovery. It were Ford et al. in 1956 (15) who showed that this effect is caused by the seeding of stem cells into a host matrix. Since then, the field has developed dramatically and one may estimate that more than a thousand leukemic patients have, by now, received a total body radiation exposure with 800 - 1200 cGy or more followed by the transfusion of allogeneic bone marrow cell suspensions, containing a sufficient number of hemopoietic stem cells to substitute for the stem cells lost by irradiation and to cause a complete hemopoietic chimera (16). Of course, this form of treatment requires a lot of detailed pathophysiological knowledge and significant efforts including the handling of genetic differences between graft and recipient, but also the spectrum of replacement therapy.

Nevertheless, it is reasonable to assume that through the advent of this new form of treatment, the value for an LD 50/30 or 60 days can - under favourable circumstances - be increased by a factor of 3 - 4.

Considering the possibilities to move the value of the LD 50 in the human
being one has to remember that only the intensive care using fluid replacement, antibiotics as well as blood cell replacement can be performed
routinely in everyone. With this form of therapy, the LD 50 value may be
modified by a factor of 1.5 or 2.0. If one wants to shift the LD 50 value
even more, then this becomes possible by hemopoietic stem cell transfusion. At this time, the bone marrow of histocompatible, if possible, related donors needs to be used (Fig. 2).

Fig.2:

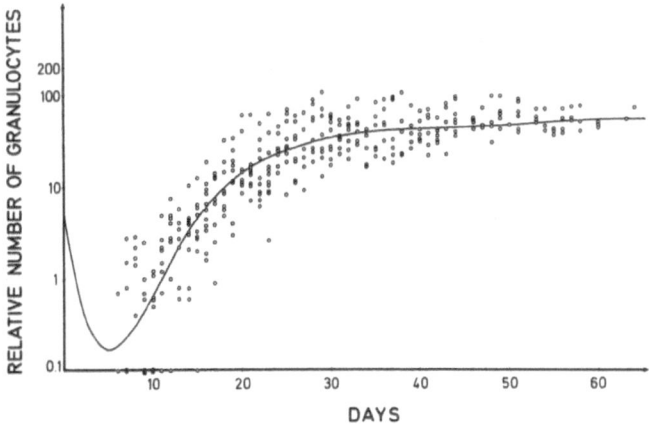

Recovery of granulocytes in patients with leukemia treated
by chemotherapy, total body irradiation and allogeneic bone
marrow transplantation. The circles on each day represent
the granulocyte concentration of one patient. The solid line
is the computer calculation based on a myelopoietic recovery
model developed in our research team.

Preclinical studies in dogs reveal, however, that this limitation may
well be overcome as time goes on. In our own team, we were able to show
that a lethally irradiated dog may be rescued if he is transfused not
only with stem cells collected from the bone marrow but also those collected from the peripheral blood and from fetal liver   (17, 18) (Fig. 3).
In the case of the use of blood derived stem cells, a large number can be
obtained by continuous flow leukocytapheresis using dextran sulfate as a
stem cell mobilizing agent. The number of cells collected in one 3-4 hour
leukocytapheresis is enough to reconstitute the bone marrow of an allogeneic recipient. This type of stem cell transplantation does not result
in a lethal graft-versus-host reaction, if a purified stem cell suspension is given in which as many as possible T- and B-cells have been
removed by gradient separation technics (19). Under certain circumstances,
it also appears possible to use stem cells from fetal liver. At the present time, this approach is only successful if the donor cells are closely
related by specific breeding to the irradiated recipient (20).

Fig. 3:

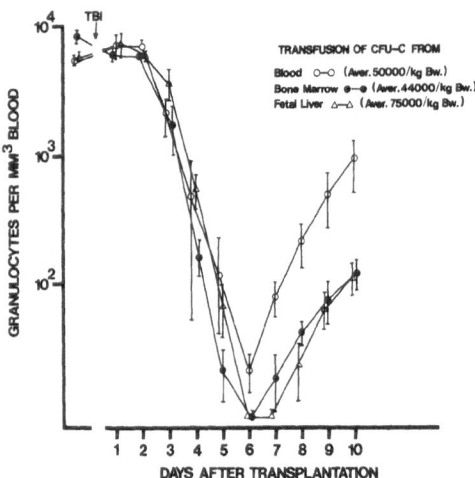

Early granulocyte recovery after total body irradiation of
dogs given mononuclear cells collected from blood, bone
marrow and fetal liver. Equal numbers of CFU-C in the suspension transfused result in slower recovery rates if bone
marrow or fetal liver are compared to blood derived progenitor cells.

5. Summary and Conclusions

.1 The survival time of mammals including man after total body exposure
to penetrating ionizing radiation is characterized by a dose-dependent reduction in the range up to about 1000 cGy, a dose-independent
3.5 or 7 day plateau at doses between about 1000 and 5000 (occasion-
ally 10 000) cGy and a dose dependent reduction above this dose. Death
in the dose range up to about 1000 cGy is correlated with hemopoietic
failure, at doses in the range from 1000 to 5000 cGy with failure of
the intestinal as well as hemopoietic cell systems and above that with
a failure of the coordinating capabilities of the CNS.

.2 This dose-effect relationship can be modified by biological factors
which include

- replacement of body fluids when severe loss occurs as a consequence of denudation of the intestinal surfaces

- complete or selected decontamination of the microbial flora of
the intestinal tract and use of professional gnotobiotic techni.'es

- selective replacement of blood cells when necessary due to imminent
functional failure

= red cells in case of anemia

= granulocytes in case of severe granulocytopenia if the administration of antibiotics is not sufficient

= platelets in case of severe thrombocytopenia

The limitation of this form of dose-response modification lies in the degree of injury to the hemopoietic stem cell pool. It is only successful as long as there is a good chance of spontaneous hemopoietic regeneration within 2 - 4 weeks after total body exposure. It may well be that the stem cell pool can regenerate spontaneously if it is not reduced to values less than 2 % of normal. This means that the LD 50 value may be modified by this form of systemic replacement therapy by a factor of 1.5 to 2.0 at the most.

.3 A further improvement can be obtained if the stem cell pool of the irradiated organism is replenished by substitution with stem cells from autologous, isogeneic or allogeneic sources. In man, the bone marrow is the conventional source at present. In animal experiments, stem cells for transplantation can also be obtained from blood as well as from fetal liver. In all these instances it can be shown that the engraftment of a sufficiently large number of stem cells from suitable donors results in a regular regeneration of hemopoiesis. Together with a prudent use of the "replacement therapies", the "stem cell substitution" may well result in a shift of the LD 50 value by a factor of 3.0 to 4.0. In other words, if the LD 50/60 days in man is considered to be in the order of 450 cGy (1), than the intensive use of modern therapeutic possibilities may well change this value under favourable circumstances to 1350 or 1800 cGy respectively.

References

1. Bond, V.P., T.M. Fliedner and J.O. Archambeau (Eds.) (1965):
   Mammalian Radiation Lethality. A Disturbance in Cellular Kinetics.
   Academic Press, New York and London

2. Matsuzawa, R. and R. Wilson:
   The intestinal mucosa of germfree mice after whole-body irradiation
   with 3 kilo roentgen.
   Radiat. Res. 25, 15-24, 1965

3. McLaughlin, M., M.P. Dacquisto, D.P. Jacobus and R.E. Horowitz:
   Effects of the Germfree State on Responses of Mice to Whole Body
   Irradiation.
   Radiat. Res. 23, 333 - 349, 1964

4. Taketa, S.T.:
   Water-electrolyte and antibiotic therapy against acute (3 to 5 day)
   intestinal radiation death in the rat.
   Radiat. Res. 16, 312-326, 1962

5. Thomas, E.D., C.A. Ashley, H.L. Lochte, A. Jaretzki III, jr., O.D.
   Sahler and J.W. Ferrebee:
   Homografts of bone marrow in dogs after lethal total-body irradiation.
   Blood 14, 720 - 736, 1959

6. Heit, H,,W. Heit, E. Kohne, T.M. Fliedner and P. Hughes:
   Allogeneic Bone Marrow Transplantation in Conventional Mice: I.
   Effect of Antibiotic Therapy on Long Term Survival of Allogeneic
   Chimaeras.
   Blut 35, 143 - 153, 1977

218

7. Kurrle, E., C. Abt, S. Bhaduri, H. Heimpel, D. Krieger, E. Vanek
and B. Kubanek:
Possibilities and Problems of Protective Isolation and Antimicrobial
Decontamination in Man.
Fliedner T.M. et al. (Eds.): Clinical and Experimental Gnotobiotics,
Zbl. Bakt. Suppl. 7, 63-66, 1979
Gustav-Fischer Verlag Stuttgart, New York

8. Freireich, E.J. et al.:
The function and fate of transfused leukocytes from donors with
chronic myelocytic leukemia in leukopenic recipients.
Ann. NY Acad. Sci. 113, 1081-1089, 1964

9. Teller, W.M. et al. (Eds.):
Rearing of non-identical twins with lymphopenic hypogammaglobulin-
aemia under gnotobiotic conditions.
Acta Paediatrica scandinavica, Suppl. 240, 1973

10. Sorensen, D.K., V.P. Bond, E.P. Cronkite and V. Perman:
An effective therapeutic regimen for the hemopoietic phase of the
acute radiation syndrome in dogs.
Radiat. Res. 13, 669-685, 1960

11. Kurrle, E., S. Bhaduri, D. Krieger, H. Pflieger and H. Heimpel:
Antimicrobial prophylaxis in acute leukemia: prospective randomized
study comparing two methods of selective decontamination.
Klin. Wochenschr. 61, 691-698, 1983

12. McCulloch, E.A. and J.E. Till:
Sensitivity of Cells from Normal Mouse Bone Marrow to Gamma Radiation
in vitro and in vivo.
Radiat. Res. 16, 822-832, 1962

13. Morley, A., E.A. King-Smith and F. Stohlman JR:
The Oscillatory Nature of Hemopoiesis.
F. Stohlman, JR (Ed.): Hemopoietic Cellular Proliferation,
3 - 14, 1970, Grune & Stratton, New York and London

14. Lorenz, E., D. Uphoff and H. Sutton:
Modification of acute irradiation injury in mice and guinea-pigs by
bone marrow injections.
Radiology 58, 863 - 877, 1952

15. Ford, C.E., J.L. Hamerton, D.W.H. Barnes and L.F. Loutit:
Cytological Identification of Radiation Chimeras.
Nature 177, 452-   , 1956

16. Gale, R.P. (Ed.):
Recent Advances in Bone Marrow Transplantation. Proceedings of the
UCLA Symposia Conference, Park City, Utah, March 13-18, 1983.
Alan R. Liss, Inc., New York, 1983

17. Raghavachar, A., O. Prümmer, T.M. Fliedner, W. Calvo, I.B.E. Stein-
    bach:
    Stem Cells from Peripheral Blood and Bone Marrow: A Comparative
    Evaluation of the Hemopoietic Potential in the Dog.
    Intern. J. of Cell Cloning 1, 191-205, 1983

18. Grilli, G., W. Calvo, F. Carbonell, M. Haen, W. Nothdurft, T.M.
    Fliedner:
    Collection, Cryopreservation and Transfusion of Fetal Liver Cells
    for the Restoration of Hemopoiesis in Lethally Irradiated Dogs.
    F. Gavosto, G.P. Bagnara, M.A.Brunelli, C.Castaldini (Eds.): Hemo-
    lymphopoiesis: Normal and Pathological Cell Differentiation,
    193 - 197, 1981
    Editrice Esculapio-Bologna

19. Körbling, M., T.M. Fliedner, W. Calvo, W.M. Ross, W. Nothdurft and
    I. Steinbach:
    Albumin Density Gradient Purification of Canine Hemopoietic Blood
    Stem Cells (HBSC): Long-Term Allogeneic Engraftment without
    GvH-Reaction.
    Exp. Hematol. 7, 277-288, 1979

20. Prümmer, O., A. Raghavachar, W. Calvo, F. Carbonell and T.M. Fliedner:
    Restoration of Hemopoiesis by Cryopreserved Fetal Liver Cells in a
    Canine Model.
    Gale, R.P. (Ed.): Recent Advances in Bone Marrow Transplantation.
    857-863, 1983
    Alan R. Liss, Inc., New York 1983

Summary of Discussions Following Presentations on Marrow Response and Hemopoietic Syndromes

James J. Conklin

Armed Forces Radiobiology Research Institute, Bethesda, Maryland, U.S.A

Canine Marrow Responses and Lethality Under Chronic Gamma Irradiation. T.M. Seed, T.E. Fritz, and D.V. Tolle.

Van Bekkum initiated the discussion by noting that the incidence of lymphoproliferative syndromes was highest in the control group. Seed noted that the incidence of lymphoproliferative diseases is acutally lower in the irradiated group in their canine population. Seed also related that no myeloproliferative disease occurred except after irradiation in the canine system. These disorders increase enormously up to 44% under the dose level of 10R per day in the canine system, resulting in fatal leukemia.

Silini observed at least two reasons for not being able to apply the Elkind Recovery to the data. The first reason is that the Elkind Recovery applies only to cell survival. Here you are not using it for cell survival. The second reason is the interpretation of the data acording to time. The population of cells that sees the first dose must be exactly the same as sees the second dose, which is not the same, because the cells continue dividing in the meantime. So, it seems that you cannot apply this type of reasoning. It also seems that you have showed that by prolonging the irradiation, you will gradually select cells that have a different type of characteristic. Seed responded that selection does play a role. Selection occurs, and it is most prominent after hematopoietic crisis. They did not see changes in radiosensitivity in the radiosensitive stage, where you place the dog in the field or the hematopoietic tissue in the field and see a gradual decline. A gradual increase is not observed in acquired radioresistance, which rules out that simple selection is the whole story here.

Seed answered in the affirmative to a question by Carsten about using tritiated thymidine suicide to measure cell proliferation in the bone marrow cells. A discussion followed, led by Carsten. He noted that you can expose mice continually to tritium. The bone marrow cellularity looks the same and everything looks normal. When you take out that bone marrow, you find you have reduced the number of CFU's (stem cells). This becomes apparent by raising the tritiated thymidine suicide level, leaving fewer CFU's to do the work of more in the G_0 state, and in this way get selection. If you look at the whole animal and the radiosensitivity, the animal may well have fewer stem cells and be more sensitive. These cells that have been brought out of a G_0 state have more radioresistance. Seed noted that they had looked at suicide-type analysis with cytosine arabinoside, but had decided to use enriched heterogeneous progenitor populations versus those that are depleted with the cells in S phase. Heterogeneous populations versus depleted populations had standard dose-response curves performed. They did not see an increase in the radiosensitivity as expected in the depleted population. If acquired radioresistance was solely responsible for the cells in S phase, it would not account for the resistance that we see later on.

222

Conklin then asked if the heart failure that was reported was secondary to hypotension, depleted intravascular volume, or a primary myocardial effect. Lemaire said that it was not studied. It was noted, however, that after irradiation, the pigs were moribund, and it was very difficult to phlebotomize the animal without hemorrhage 2 or 3 days after exposure. Conklin suggested that it was depleted intravascular volume for a number of reasons. First, capillary permeability is markedly increased in the gut and in the pulmonary parenchyma. Second, the venous system dilates, particularly in the mesenteric circulation. In a number of studies done at AFRRI by Hawkins, Doyle, and Cockerham, significant venous pooling in the gut has been shown. Third, there is also significant dilation in the vascular bed of the skin. Finally, in some experiments where canines were bilaterally irradiated with 6,000, 8,000, and 10,000 rads selectively to the myocardium, normal cardiac performance was seen until somewhere between 45 to 90 days later. He concluded that the acute changes were all peripheral, pulmonary, or mesenteric vascular derangements plus hemorrhage that were causing their problems.

Radiation Syndromes, LD 50 and RBE of Neutrons. J.J. Broerse.

Ainsworth began the discussion by noting that he had always been intrigued by the fact that Broerse's extrapolation number for the in vitro CFU survival curve was different from the extrapolation number for the in vivo survival curve, and that the D_o was also different. Broerse replied that one of the aspects that had not yet been explained was a difference in scoring the response with a delay, and comparing the day after the neutron irradiation to the day after photon irradiation. Ainsworth asked why Broerse expected it to be different. Some people find different answers, and some people don't. Both kinds of observations exist in the literature. The extrapolation number is 1-1.5 for X-rays while Broerse reports 3-4 for X-rays. Others find very little difference in the extrapolation number. Silini commented that he would emphasize the in vivo data, and there the extrapolation number is 2.5.

Kaul asked for clarification of the dosimetry on the mice. Unilateral exposure of the mice, even with some reasonably high energy photons, would produce a gradient in a mouse. He asked what doses were recorded. Broerse answered that there was not time enough in the morning session to go into all of the details. The mice were always irradiated under conditions of maximum backscatter. Then the dose distribution over the animal was better than explained in the a.m. session by Zoetelief.

Fliedner noted that it is important to take into consideration the density of ionization in the bone marrow itself. Fliedner related that at lower and lower dose rates, Feinendegen has pointed out that you spare some stem cells. You have to deal with a very complex system of stem cell pools that are feedback-regulated. Many years ago it was pointed out that the CFU's of the repopulating cell go down (let's say at the dose of 16 R per day) to about 10% of normal, while the iron incorporation remains completely normal after an initial decrease. That indicates that the maintenance of this hemopoiesis is from a former mature level at the cost of the reduced pluripotent stem cell, which means that the whole system is turning over faster. Fritz responded that this view was not suported by what Dr. Seed shows in the suicide techniques, because it does not kill any more cells than he does in the normal population. Yet the response is equally different when he does the cell-survival curve. That curve is fairly stable over a long period of time. After 2000 hours of radiation, it maintains a steady state; so whether he irradiates now or later, he has the same kinetics. It does not support the idea of a more rapid turnover. Fliedner noted that Seed et al. measured only GM-CFC. Fritz acknowledged that the GM-CFC is something completely different from the pluripotent stem cell.

Hematopoietic Syndrome of Pigs. G. Lemaire and J. Maas.

Broerse began the discussion of this paper with a question about neutron dosimetry and the use of sulfur pellets. He noted that Lemaire used beta-induced activity of the P-32 to measure the dose. In his earlier work, Broerse compared the sulphur activation with ionization chambers, and found no problems with 14-MeV neutrons. As neutron energy decreased, the cross sections changed considerably and resulted in discrepancies. Broerse emphasized that the activation method should be complemented by ionization chambers. Lemaire replied that the sulfur activation studies were used to correlate with ionization chambers.

Smith asked if histopathologic studies of the gastrointestinal tract were performed. Lemaire related that only macroscopic examinations were performed, which showed diffuse hemorrhage in many internal organs. Conklin commented that during atmospheric testing, 1-year-old miniature pigs were exposed to a mixed field of 400 rads of neutrons and photons. They had profound gastrointestinal derangement, showing submucosal hemorrhage, pseudomembrane formation, edema, and sloughing of the mucous membrane.

Broerse's group can get a value that is representative of the average dose over the animal. He noted that he had studied the cells at the bone-soft tissue interface. They have never taken the trouble to try to identify these cells since they need a model of the location of the most sensitive hemopoietic stem cells and where they are located. Kaul remarked that it is interesting that when you are comparing the photon and the neutron differences, there is no way you could actually do a site-dependent assay. If everything could be stopped for a moment, you might actually see (especially with neutrons) more of a gradient with the neutrons than with the photons, and more of a gradient with the 250-KeV X-ray than with the cesium gamma rays. When you correlate everything in terms of a single value, even with a mouse, the number that you are correlating has difficulties. That is the problem of dealing with just a single number of merit.

Broerse replied that, for the monkeys, they begin as closely to ideal conditions as possible. This means that they rotate the monkey in front of the converter plate inside the reactor, and rotate the monkey in front of the X-ray machine. These depth-dose patterns are then closely comparable for the 300-KeV X-ray and for the fission neutron. Broerse felt that what was seen is really a difference in the radiation sensitivity dose survival curves, which are now known for different systems and are different because of intrinsic differences in radiosensitivity. Kaul reiterated that this could also explain the issue of why a different D_o is seen in vitro and in vivo. In vitro there is fairly unambiguous dosimetry, whereas in vivo it is somewhat more ambigious. The two numbers are not the same, and they don't become the same number until you get to very high photon energies. Only under those circumstances can you make a direct comparison. Silini remarked that, to a biologist, they will be second-degree types of differences, which formerly had not been looked at. He did not look into this problem and Broerse did not look into this, because it is not the primary interest in establishing mechanisms for the pathogenesis of the disease.

Young stated that he wanted to reinforce what Broerse had said. In his study with monkeys at the NRL cyclotron using high-energy neutrons and a matched bremsstrahlung field, a miniature ionization chamber was used to map the field across the monkey's head. The dose to mid-head was also mapped all the way across the field. The inverse square law was used to get the same depth-dose distribution for bremsstrahlung as for the high-energy neutrons. When he calculated the LD-50/5 for the animals, he obtained an RBE value of 1.4. Ainsworth added that when he did a 400-dog study in 1963-65, in terms of midline-tissue dose exposure, they saw an RBE of 1.3. The mean survival time of the neutron radiation was appreciably shorter than for the reactor gamma. This led to the belief that there was some gamma contribution to the depth damage at the LD-50/30 in the neutron-irradiated dog. They also did a 14-MeV neutron dog study in which the LD-50 was higher than expected compared to fission neutron.

Response of Man to Accidental Irradiation. K.F. Baverstock.

The discussion of Baverstock's paper was begun by Fliedner, who asked what is wrong with the doses that he published in the 1965 book (1). He asked if Baverstock had consulted and checked what is wrong with the dose calculations that Broerse and others did at that time? Baverstock responded that he had not. He noted that there was such a wide range of doses, and identified uncertainties that should be acknowledged. Fliedner noted that biologically there was really no difference in the response of the hemopoietic system between the Vinca and the Oak Ridge accident (where he was present at the time of the accident). In the Vinca and Oak Ridge situations, the data showed that the hemopoietic system in the two groups of people reacted almost the same with regard to rate of regeneration and onset of regeneration.

Kaul asked why there had been no attempt to analytically recreate geom- etry and map the location where people were at the time the accident occurred. Baverstock responded that individual A claimed to have been at a particular point at the time of the accident. From his position and from the number of fissions that were to have taken place in the drum at the time, it was thought that he had a dose of around 1000-2000 rems. Clearly he did not.

Kaul noted that the evidence presented indicated that the hematopoietic depression at 30 days was actually higher for the accident with the smallest dose. The data also showed only two orientations, an anterior and a side. He asked if no one was facing away. You will get the maximum dose to the marrow from a posterior and not a side exposure. Baverstock replied that to account for the sodium-24 in the blood, he had to be closer to the reactor to get that level of sodium-24.

Vriesendorp raised a question about large-animal models in which the hemopoietic stem cell is not the dose-limiting cell. He was surprised by the Argonne experience that, even at these extreme dose rates, the bone marrow always seemed to remain the dose-limiting tissue. Fliedner answered the question by noting the fibrotic changes in some organs. In principle, the data suggest that human beings could survive up to 2000 or 3000 rad. The reality shows that it becomes very difficult because the gastrointestinal tract and other organs such as the lung, develop lethal complications. Vriesendorp asked the workshop members which system becomes dose limiting after bone marrow, and if there are any circumstances in which another tissue is dose limiting. Fliedner re- plied that the Asian turtle can stand kilorads, and, if it does die, it dies when it is hibernating. It does not die from the gastrointestinal symptom; it dies from lack of energy. It just lacks oxygen supply to the liver. Carsten responded that there are three limiting systems: the hemopoietic, gastrointestinal, and central nervous sytems. He also noted that Casserett has suggested that the stress-protecting mechanism (which may includes interplay between the pituitary, hypothalamus, and adrenal) may not be functioning. In very young animals, these systems may be limiting with whole-body irradiation, but in the young adult, it is the gut. Fliedner countered that from human experience, we have very rare examples of true homogeneous irradiation; consequently, the gut may become a critical organ. In the Vinca case, the critical organ was the gut. In the LA 2, it was the cardiovascular system. Finally, Carsten related that, in the first ten cases reported by Hempleman (Ann. Int.

Med. 36:279-510, 1952), the accident victims' courses were described in great detail. Not one of them had a truly uniform exposure other than perhaps the one who died immediately. In all of these you could see it was not uniform. All the pictures showed a nonuniform exposure, and they probably had plenty of bone marrow left in some parts of the body.

Smith requested a point of clarification from the Chairman. He asked if it was being suggested that if you have a man exposed to between 5 and 10 gray of whole-body radiation that his chances of survival are enhanced if he is injected or transfused with purified stem cells from blood rather than from bone marrow. Fliedner replied that he had not suggested that in his presentation. He suggested that few investigators addressed what they would actually do with patients in the dose range (500 to 1000 rads). He would personally treat them as you would aplastic anemia, including pretreatment with cyclophosphamide. He felt this was neccessry with 500 to 1000 rad because they may not have complete immunosuppression. Van Bekkum countered that there was no evidence in humans that putting in bone marrow might worsen the situation. In mice, greater mortality is obtained if you do not treat the donor bone marrow. What should we do with people in the midlethal dose range? There is evidence that this phenomenon does not occur in large animals, so he would just infuse bone marrow without preconditioning with cyclophosphamide. If there is sufficient marrow left, the marrow can be rejected and the patient can recover. If there aren't enough residual stem cells, the marrow will probably help. Vriesendorp was asked his opinion about midlethal dose exposures and how to treat those patients. He replied that it would depend on two factors: (1) the amount of immune suppression given by the accidental irradiation, and (2) the type of donor available, whether it is an HLA-identical donor or a twin. He would try to follow the bone marrow transplant protocol to get the graft going optimally. Fliedner observed that there was one good example in the Mol case where the patient had a very inhomogeneous exposure. The highest dose was in the leg and pelvic region, and fortunately Jaimet waited rather than transplant. At 12 days he saw the typical hematopoietic rebound and regeneration when he punctured the cervical spinous process and found active marrow. So that was a good indication that there was enough inhomogeneity to repopulate the entire marrow by the migration of the stem cells from these intact areas.

Kaul asked a question about some of the Vinca patients relative to the hemograms. A point was made that after reaching a nadir, the two Oak Ridge patients and the Vinca patients behaved the same way; yet it is very clear that before that point, they did not behave the same way. It was mentioned that this could be due to low-energy neutrons producing a gradient at Vinca. Kaul speculated that from what was presented it looks more like a gradient at Oak Ridge. Were there sufficient neutrons to make such a gradient important? This seems to be more or less substantiated by the fact that it was the uniformity of exposure at Vinca that gave a uniformly low initial hemogram, whereas the gradient at Oak Ridge gave a gradually decreasing hemogram. Because of the small amount of marrow that survived and could not support itself, it subsequently went to the minimum. This would lead to exactly the opposite conclusion that Fliedner initially reached. Fliedner responded that the whole system has to be considered as a feedback-regulated system. If you give lower radiation doses, your recovery is much slower. When you irradiate the stem cell pool (100%) and decrease it to a fraction of normal, you have at least two stem cell populations left. One population is intact, and complete replication can occur. The other population is injured, but the feedback regulator factor does not recognize that this is actually a partially perturbed stem cell population. Initially, the body will act as if this is the entire population from which regeneration occurs. The fact is (the data are in agreement) that only the unperturbed pool permits final recovery. The problem is that none of us, even with the best retrospective analysis, can know what the stem cell fraction is, regardless of the quality of radiation. The relationship between the partially injured stem cell population and the complete and intact population really makes the difference in the kinetics of regeneration.

Silini added that what is quite clear from mouse experience is that the way the system behaves depends entirely on the fraction of stem cells that are complete and intact. Conklin noted that there were very few early hematologic data in the Vinca accident. The most noticeable case was in the lymphocytes. Lymphocyte counts were not done until 48 hours, whereas the most profound derangements in lymphocytes occur in the first 24 to 48 hours. The curve that was plotted shows that all the lymphocytes started at a much lower baseline. If the first hemograms were not performed until 48 hours, that is exactly where those curves should start, because later they have essentially the same slopes and recovery is the same. Fliedner responded that he never put much attention to the absolute values because they were not done in the same laboratory, but that the slopes were important.

SUMMARY OF ROUND TABLE DISCUSSION ON RESPONSE OF
DIFFERENT SPECIES

J.J. Broerse and T.J. MacVittie
Radiobiological Institute TNO, Rijswijk, the Netherlands and
Armed Forces Radiobiological Research Institute,
Bethesda, Maryland, U.S.A.

In preparing the workshop the organizers formulated a number of
key questions which were considered to be of great relevance to the
subject. Under the chairmanship of van Bekkum the following four i-
tems were covered during the round table discussion:

1. Standardization of dosimetry and experimental procedures

To allow a comparison of biological results obtained by various
groups a common basis for dosimetry and experimental arrangements is
essential. The different institutes studying the acute effects of radiation in larger animals have employed various more or less realistic
phantoms. Broerse mentioned that for studies in rodents, a dosimetry
protocol and a code of practice are in preparation (J. Zoetelief, R.W.
Davies and J.J. Broerse, EULEP protocol for X-ray dosimetry, Commission of the European Communities, 1984), however this has not yet
been established for dogs, monkeys or miniature pigs. MacVittie and
Kaul emphasized the need to provide sufficient information on source
characteristics in a quantitative and qualitative way. To derive the absorbed dose in different organs in retrospect it will further be important to report the mass of the animal, its orientation and the entrance
midline and exit absorbed dose. Kaul stated that it would be valuable
to set up a data base on dose distributions in various phantoms in dependence on the energy and angular distribution of the incident photon radiation. Van Bekkum questioned the usefulness of data bases
since there is generally no selection on the input. Kaul replied that a
good data base has been established for the dosimetry of the Hiroshima
and Nagasaki atomic bomb survivors but had to admit that the costs
for this operation exceeded one million dollars. Considering the present
limited availability of research funds, Silini and van Bekkum would not
put their priorities on expensive dosimetry programs for acute radiation effects but would prefer to support research in other areas including radiation carcinogenesis.

2. Extrapolation of LD_{50} values for unilateral irradiation from information for homogeneous standardized conditions.

MacVittie wanted to know the relevancy of bilateral uniform exposure data to extrapolate to a crude endpoint such as LD_{50} over 5 or
30 days when the exposure is unilateral and restricted to part of the

body since this is the population the physicians will see following a nuclear disaster. Carsten commented that soldiers should wear dosimetry badges at different sides of their body. After accidental exposure, read-out of the dosimeters will allow an estimation of the absorbed dose received and determine the possibilities for medication of the radiation victims.

Ainsworth mentioned his studies with dogs where the $LD_{50/30}$ values after 1 MVP X-irradiations were increased by 20 percent for unilateral irradiation as compared with bilateral irradiation. For the irradiation with fission neutrons he did not observe a change in LD_{50} for these two exposure conditions. Conklin reminded the audience about the results of Schick et al (reported at the RSG 5 NATO meeting, Paris, april 1981) who showed that shielding of different parts of the body results in an increase by a factor of 3 in the LD_{50} for mice with reference to whole body irradiation. According to Conklin this finding is of great practical importance since inhomogeneous exposures (e.g. due to shielding of the pelvis) can be envisaged inside military vehicles and aircrafts.

Returning to the effects of unilateral irradiations Fliedner critized the use of LD_{50} values as a baseline for comparison of different exposures. He strongly suggested to use a functional endpoint since in each species the reason for dying at the LD_{50} level is different. In some animals it will be anemia, in others it can be platelet depression or granulocytopenia and infection. Smith mentioned his work at Harwell where they measure dicentric aberrations in lymphocytes after culture as a biological indicator for radiation damage. With these techniques they can determine doses in the range from 0.1 to 3 Gy. The limitation of the technique is that it cannot detect nonuniform exposures. The yield of dicentric aberrations can only be expressed in terms of total body equivalent dose, however at present they try to make the technique also applicable for nonuniform irradiations. Van Bekkum considered this to be an interesting approach under normal laboratory conditions but questioned its usefulness in an emergency situation when thousands of people would have been exposed. In this connection Carsten recommended the use of cytogenetic tests including sister-chromatid exchanges, scoring of micronuclei and examination of biochemical parameters of haemotopoietic stem cells. He further stated the need for a better understanding of stromal factors in defining radiosensitivity.

In summarizing this part of the discussion van Bekkum, Fliedner and Silini underlined that the relevant parameters determining the radiation response are the number of functional stem cells. When infections are considered the number of granulocytes during the first 10 days after exposure are important; for haemorrhages it is the number of thrombocytes. The emphasis should not be placed on the actual number of stem cells (static concept) but on the number of functional differentiated cells that can be produced by these stem cells (dynamic concept).

3. Correlation between tissue specific lethality and inactivation of the functional stem cells.

Van Bekkum called attention to the fact that studies on chemical protection of animals, the effects of anoxia and the RBE of fast neutrons (as reported by Broerse) all agree perfectly with the D_0 values of haemopoietic stem cells. On the contrary Krebs and Jones (Radiation Research 51, 374-380, 1972) concluded that a difference in dose rate producing a large difference in LD_{50} is not necessarily associated with a corresponding difference in response of the haemopoietic stem cells. Van Bekkum had checked this reference and formulated two points of criticism. In the first place the ratio of the LD_{50} values for high and low dose rates (873 and 1359 R respectively) is not much different from that for the lowest D_0 value of 82R (95% confidence limits) at the high dose rate and the highest D_0 value of 118 R at low dose rate. Secondly he argued that the experiment of Krebs and Jones was not well designed. The irradiations at high and low dose rates involved total exposure times of 30 minutes and 7 hours, respectively. During the latter exposure time there will be repair of radiation damage and repopulation of functional cells. The D_0 values were all derived from irradiation with a maximum exposure of 500 R i.e. a maximum irradiation time of 2 1/2 hours. In consequence van Bekkum concluded that these D_0 values are not valid for calculating the surviving fraction of colony forming cells after a 7 hour exposure. The results of Krebs and Jones do not disprove the idea that haemopoietic stem cells are the baseline for the LD_{50} levels.

Ainsworth stated that the D_0 values of stem cells and LD_{50} agree for an unperturbed hematopoietic system but that this not the case when the haemopoiesis has been perturbed by prior irradiation. Fliedner warned the audience that one should not speak about a direct correlation. Due to feedback mechanisms and the sigmodial shape of dose response curves, the survival of stem cells and the occurrence of the bone marrow syndrome are not linearly correlated.

4. RBE for occurrence of bone marrow syndrome after irradiation with gamma rays and megavoltage X rays.

Broerse introduced this item by stating that sometimes the choice of dose levels for high energy photons are based on the clinical experience with conventional X rays. For the occurrence of the bone marrow syndrome in mice he and Zoetelief observed an average RBE of 0,86 for ^{137}Cs gamma-rays, however this was not always confirmed by other investigators. Deviations of 10 percent in absorbed dose will induce considerable differences in biological response. Consequently it will be important to establish an RBE for haemopoietic death in larger species including man after exposure to high energy photons. Vriesendorp reported his experiments at Chicago on bone marrow transplantation in dogs after irradiation with ^{60}Co gamma rays. For the acute toxicity (bone marrow syndrome) and immunosuppression he observed an RBE of 0.9 with reference to 200 kV X rays. Vriesendorp was unable to quote an RBE for the induction of late effects. Fliedner stressed the importance of looking at individual cell populations (e.g. lymphocyte counts) when comparing different photon energies.

At the end of the round table discussion Silini inquired about the dosimetric value of functional tests performed in France notably electroencephalograms in accidentally irradiated people. Lemaire confirmed that Court, Bagot and coworkers at Fontenay-aux-Roses have observed perturbations in the EEG after irradiations with doses as low as 0.4 Gy. (Their studies on monkeys and rabbits were reported at the RSG 5 NATO meeting, Paris, april 1981).

Finally Silini asked attention for the problem in how far the radiation response can be predicted. Fliedner mentioned the competition between differentiation and replication. He stated that there is no single prognostic factor but emphasized the need of day to day scoring of functional cells. Vriesendorp considered the study of the dynamic behaviour of stem cells during 5 to 6 days post irradiation a retrospective test. When you have assessed the loss of regeneration the patients will die anyhow from bone marrow aplasia. Fliedner did not agree and stated that even after twelve hours the prognosis becomes more clear. Carsten felt that there is a need for more accurate measurements of the distribution of active bone marrow cells in the human. These statements concluded a very lively and stimulating workshop on the response of different species to high dose total body irradiation.

SUBJECT INDEX